The Big Book Of Essential Oil Recipes For Beauty

Over 200 Homemade Aromatherapy Essential Oil Recipes For All-Round Natural Body Care

MEL HAWLEY

ISBN-13: 978-1537767536

ISBN-10: 1537767534

DEDICATION

All things bright and beautiful

All creatures great and small

All things wise and wonderful

The Lord God made them all

TABLE OF CONTENTS

INTRODUCTION 1

   Essential Oils & Beauty 1

   Other Books By Mel Hawley 3

BODY SCRUB RECIPES 4

   Basic Sugar Scrub... 5

   Citrus Coffee Scrub 5

   Spicy Sugar Scrub.. 6

   Rosemary Mint 7

   Magnesium Winter Scrub... 7

   Soothing Brown Sugar Scrub 8

   Grapefruit/ Sugar Scrub... 9

   Cinnamon Vanilla Body Scrub... 9

   Spicy Oat 10

   Lemon Milk Sugar 11

   Oatmeal &Peels 12

   Peppermint Citrus.. 12

   Chamomile Petitgrain 13

   Honey Herb Scrub.. 13

   Vanilla Patchouli 14

   Peppermint-Citrus Salt Scrub 15

BATH RECIPES 16

BATH SALTS... 16

   Margarita Bath Salt.. 17

   Aromatherapy Bath Salts... 17

Seaside Bath Salt Soak 18

Lemon Bath Salt.. 19

Oatmeal, Milk And Honey Salt Bath 20

Natural Grapefruit Bath Salts 21

Ocean Bath Salts... 22

Rose-Scented Bath Salts 23

BATH BOMB RECIPES 24

No- Citrus Acid Bath Bombs.. 24

Scented Bath Bombs.. 25

Fizzy Bath Bombs 26

Cane Sugar Bath Bombs.. 27

Dried Flower Bath Bombs 28

Peppermint Bath Bombs... 29

Minty Eucalyptus Bath Bombs.. 30

Goat's Milk Bath Bombs 31

Rooibos Detox Bombs.. 31

Dried Flower Bath Bombs 32

Lavender & Oatmeal Bath Bombs 33

BATH OILS 35

Simple Aromatherapy Bath Oil 35

Blissful Oil Bath 36

Muscle Relaxing Bath Oil Blend 36

Sensuous Oil Bath 37

Revitalizing Oil Bath 37

Relaxing Oil Bath 38

Shampoo Bath Oil 39

Lavender Soothing Bath Oil 40

Soothing Aromatherapy Bath Oil 40

Alcohol Bath Oil 41

BUBBLE BATH RECIPES 43

Citrus Sunshine Bubble Bath 43

Lavender Uplifting Bubble Bath 44

Silky And Spicy Bubble Bath 45

Rose Absolute Bubble Bath 46

Sweet Vanilla Bubble Bath 47

MILK BATH RECIPES 48

Plain Milk Bath 48

Skin Softening Milk Bath 49

Sweet Vanilla Milk Bath 49

Meadow Milk Bath 50

Lavender Milk Bath 51

Spicy And Silky Milk Bath 51

Rose Absolute Milk Bath 52

BATH TEAS & OTHER RECIPES 54

Relaxing Bath Tea 54

Green Herbal Bath Tea 55

Oatmeal Herbal Bath Tea 56

SHOWER STEAMER RECIPES 57

Revitalizing Shower Steamer 57

Anti-Stuffiness Shower Steamer 59

After Workout Shower Steamer 60

Elevating Shower Steamer 62

Relaxing Shower Steamer 63

Spicy Shower Steamer 65

Easy Homemade Shower Gel 66

Lavender & Chamomile Bath Melts 67

FACIAL STEAMS RECIPES 69

Facial Steam For Normal And Combination Skin 69

Facial Steam For Mature, Dry And Sensitive Skin 70

Facial Steam For Acne And Oily Skin 71

FACIAL MASKS RECIPES 73

Essential Oil Blackhead Removal Mask 73

Face Mask For Normal Skin 74

Face Mask For Dry And Mature Skin 75

Turmeric Face Mask 76

Face Mask For Acne And Oily Skin 77

Acne Scar Face Mask 78

Face Mask For Sensitive And Problem Skin 79

MASSAGE OIL RECIPES 81

Sweet And Spicy Aphrodisiac Massage Oil 81

Blissful Citrus Massage Oil 82

Lavender Massage Oil 83

Lavender Massage Oil 84

Stress Relief Aromatherapy Massage Oil 85

Anti-Snoring Massage Oil 86

FACIAL SKIN TONERS RECIPES 87

Facial Skin Toner For Normal And Combination Skin 87

Facial Skin Toner For Mature, Dry And Sensitive Skin 88

Facial Skin Toner For Acne And Oily Skin.................................... 89

FACIAL SCRUBS RECIPES 90

Facial Scrub For Normal And Combination Skin 90

Facial Scrub For Dry, Mature And Damaged Skin 92

Scrub For Acne And Oily Skin.. 93

SOAP RECIPES 95

Silky Body Wash.. 95

Homemade Lemon Soap 96

Hand Wash Liquid Soap 96

Seaweed Soap... 97

Antibacterial & Antiviral Hand Wash Soap.............................. 98

Sweet Honey Soap 99

Lavender Soap 100

Simple Soap Recipe... 100

Herbal Soap 101

Basic Lotion Bars... 101

Lemon/ Cedar Men's Body Wash 102

Super Aromatic Men's Body Wash 102

Sweet & Strong Men's Body Wash 103

HAIR CARE RECIPES.. 104

Avocado Hair Moisturizing 104

Homemade Hair Softener/ Growth 105

Lavender/ Rosemary Hair Spray 106

Split Ends Remedy 107

Warm Oil Recipe For Dry Hair... 107

Itchy Scalp Shampoo Recipe 108

After Shampooing Rinse: For Dry Hair 109

Sweet-Smelling Herbal Shampoo 109

Henna Protein Treatment 110

Deep Endings Essential Oil Treatment 111

Dry Scalp Remedy With Rosemary Oil 112

Lavender Mist 113

Homemade Hair Conditioner Oil 113

Scaly Scalp And Dandruff Blend 114

Scented Hair Gel 114

Quality Hair Treatment 115

LIPS AND MOUTH CARE RECIPES 116

Pomegranate Lip Balm 116

Honey Cocoa Lip Balm 117

Honey Balm 118

Peppermint Lip Balm 118

Natural Teeth Whitener 119

Natural Toothpaste 120

Lavender Lemon Lip Balm 120

Tangerine Lip Gloss 121

Lemon Lip Gloss 122

Hemp Oil Lip Balm 122

Rose-Coco Lip Balm 123

Minty Choc Lip Balm 124

Sweet Lavender Lip Balm 125

Cold Sores Treatment Lip Balm 126

Sweet Sugar Lip Balm 127

Luscious Lip Balm 128

NAIL CARE RECIPES 129

Nail Growth Soak 129

Nail Moisturizing Soak 130

Anti-Aging Hand Oil 130

DEODORANTS AND POWDERS 132

Simple Deodorant Powder 132

Pineapple Deodorant Powder 133

Scented Orange Deodorant Powder...................................... 133

Fine Thyme Deodorant Powder.. 134

Face Powder Foundation 135

Homemade Probiotic Deodorant 135

Herbal Deodorant Powder.. 136

Sage Deodorizing Powder.. 137

Fairy Dusting Powder.. 138

Lemony Deodorant 139

Simply Fresh Deodorant Powder 140

LOTION, SHEA BUTTER AND OIL RECIPES 141

Non-Greasy Moisturizing Lotion... 142

Uplifting Homemade Lotion 143

Easy Lotion... 144

Coconut &Tamanu Body Butter.. 145

Skin Toning Body Butter 146

Lavender Makeup Setting Spray... 147

Essential Oil Blend For Baggy Eyes 148

Stretch Mark Oil... 148

Lush Body Oil 149

Orange Chocolate Body Butter 149

Homemade Sunburn Spray 150

Soothing Body Butter 151

Spot Beater Oil 152

Lime Coconut Body Butter 152

Healing Body Butter 153

Anti Cellulite Body Butter 154

Sunscreen Lotion 154

Foot Lotion For Aching Feet 156

CREAMS 157

Frankincense & Shea Butter Eye Cream 157

Beeswax Hand Cream 158

Homemade Shaving Cream 159

Rose Beeswax Hand Cream 160

Bee Pollen Hand Cream 160

Lemon Facial Cleansing Cream 161

Beeswax Cold Cream 162

Rash Cream With Aloe & Lavender 163

Beeswax Almond Hand Cream 164

Heavy Duty Hand Cream 165

DIY Stretch Mark Cream 166

Homemade Anti-Aging Serum 167

Eye Serum For Dark Circles &Puffiness 167

Moisturizing Anti-Aging Face Cream 168

Witch Hazel Eye Solution 169

PERFUMES RECIPES 170

    Whispering Drops Perfume 172

    Rich Spicy Cologne 173

    Fiery Passions Perfume.. 173

    Musky floral Perfume Blend 174

    Fruitwood Perfume.. 175

    Exotic Perfume Blend 176

    Soothing Body Perfume 177

    Summer Sweet Perfume.. 177

    Homemade Deodorant For Men 178

    Midnight Garden 179

    Love Tonic Perfume 180

    Forestry Perfume... 181

    Surprise Perfume... 181

    Tangerine -Patchouli Solid Perfume 182

    Citrus Cologne... 183

    Alpha Male Cologne... 184

    Homemade Oil Aftershave 184

    Timeout Blend 185

    Citrus Lavender Solid Perfume 187

INTRODUCTION

Essential Oils & Beauty

Using essential oils, together with other natural ingredients is one of the best things you can do for your skin. Essential oils are good for your skin because they kill bacteria, viruses and fungi, thereby making your skin germ-free. We must be mindful of the skin and body care products we regularly apply. Beauty products, with their chemical components, affect us beyond skin level. From shampoo, soap, and shaving cream to lipstick, cleansers and perfumes; commercial beauty products are filled with synthetic ingredients that are detrimental to our health.

If you take time to read the list of ingredients on the skincare products you have been using, you will discover many chemicals with complex long names. Several of these chemicals have negative effects on your skin and even your health .We need to choose a natural approach to cosmetics; and essential oil provides that alternative. Extracted from plants, bark, roots, wood, flowers or seeds, essential oils are natural, highly concentrated oils with powerful antioxidant properties. You can use them to clear up acne, reduce or eliminate wrinkles, heal your body and revitalize your hair. These botanical substances have so much to offer in the area of natural skin care.

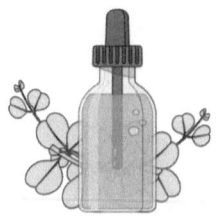

We cannot do without skin care products because as we advance in age, our skin reduces the natural oil it generates. Lotions and creams for instance, augment the skin's protective barrier when it is applied. This way, the skin loses less water through evaporation, making it feel smoother and softer. However, with essential oils, you can create lots of beauty products to keep the skin soft and healthy. Essential oils penetrate the skin easily. Within a few minutes, they are carried all through the blood and tissues where they offer tremendous therapeutic and purifying benefits.

This book is a compilation of beauty products and recipes that will enable you enjoy the benefits of natural body and skincare. The essential oils that are used in each recipe have been chosen specifically because they are the most suited for the exact purpose. However, there are some important things you must know about essential oil before starting. Consequently, I would advice that you get a copy of my first book: *The Big Book of Essential Oil Recipes for Healing & Health*. It contains lots of helpful information on essential oils as well as a wide range of recipes on healing and health.

A Few Essential Oil Tips To Remember:

- Do not use internally.
- Do not apply directly on your skin but dilute with carrier oil.
- Keep out children's reach.
- Avoid contact with eyes.
- Use only pure essential oils; stay away from synthetic fragrances.
- To avoid degradation and rancidity, store essential oils properly.
- Before experimenting with any oil, try to know its properties, precautions and dose.
- Do not use on children, pregnant women and the elderly.

Other Books By Mel Hawley

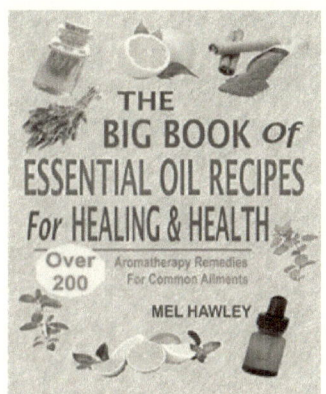

The Big Book Of Essential Oil Recipes For Healing & Health: Over 200
Aromatherapy Remedies For Common Ailments

BODY SCRUB RECIPES

Body scrubs are just great! They work by removing old layers of dead skin, leaving you with a fresh, glowing and healthy skin. This process is known as exfoliating. Additionally, they detoxify the body, help to fight cellulite and stimulate the circulation of blood and lymph. Exfoliating is crucial if you are battling acne. Using a body scrub before other skin treatments opens up the pores and makes it easier for other products to work more effectively.

The good news is that nature has blessed us with a vast array of organic and healthy ingredients such as essential oils, base oils, sugars, salts and oats to make our own natural scrubs; therefore, we need not resort to commercial body scrubs that contain dangerous chemicals which can damage the skin in the long run. There are two major types of body scrubs: salt and sugar. Salt will sting if you have scratches, or rashes. Sugar scrubs are gentler on the skin and also non-stinging so they are ideal for sensitive or irritated skin.

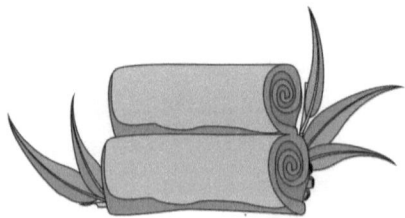

Body Scrubs - Dos And Don'ts

- Do not use body scrubs on sunburned, damaged or broken skin.
- Do not use on genitals.
- Do not allow water to get in your scrubs as it will cause the growth of mold. Store in air-tight jars in a cool, dry place.
- Do not use glass containers in the bathroom so they don't slip and break, use plastic containers instead.

- Discard scrubs with rancid smells or visible signs of molds.
- Use body scrubs (exfoliate) twice a week.

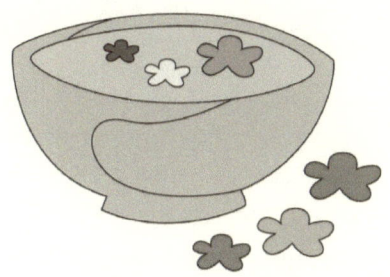

Recipes

Basic Sugar Scrub
Ingredients:

2 cups organic white sugar

1 cup carrier oil of choice

2-3 drops essential oil of choice

Citrus Coffee Scrub
Ingredients

1 cup coconut oil, melted

1 cup coffee grounds

1-3 drops orange essential oil

1-3 drops lemon essential oil

½ cup coconut sugar

Directions

1. Mix all ingredients in a bowl until thoroughly.

2. Keep at room temperature, use and store leftover in a mason jar.

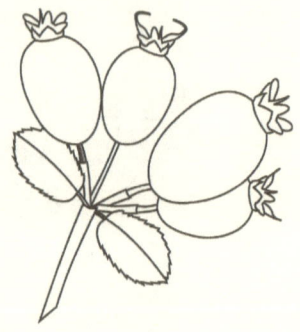

Spicy Sugar Scrub

Ingredients

1 cup sugar

2 tsp ground cloves

1 cup sesame oil

1 tsp rose essential oil

2 tsp grated orange zest

Directions

1. Mix all ingredients well.

2. Transfer the now gritty paste to an air tight container using a spoon.

3. Label, date and store in a cool place.

4. Use scrub within 3 months.

Rosemary Mint

Ingredients:

2 cups Sugar

1 cup Coconut oil

1 teaspoon Peppermint essential oil

1 teaspoon Rosemary essential oil

Directions:

1. Combine all the ingredients so it forms a paste.

2. Use a spoon to transfer mixture to an air -tight jar.

3. Label jar, date and store it in a cool and place.

Magnesium Winter Scrub

Ingredients

1 cup Epsom salt

¼ cup almond oil or olive oil

1 tsp liquid castile soap

10-15 drops peppermint and citrus essential oils

Note:

Epsom salts kelps to purify and beautify the skin, making it look beautiful, youthful and soft.

Directions

1. Mix all ingredients together in a small bowl.

2. Add essential oils until desired fragrance is achieved.

3. Store in an airtight jar.

4. Use a teaspoon sized amount to exfoliate body as needed.

5. Rinse after use. Use within 3 months.

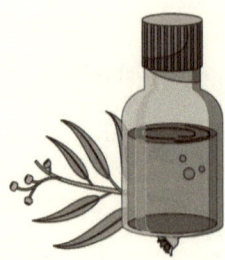

Soothing Brown Sugar Scrub

Ingredients

1 cup brown sugar

½ tsp rosewood essential oil

½ cup almond oil

½ tsp lavender essential oil

Directions

1. Mix all the ingredients together until it is paste-like.

2. Transfer to an air -tight container.

3. Store it in a cool and place.

Grapefruit/ Sugar Scrub

Ingredients:

3 drops essential oil

1/2 cup organic brown sugar

2 teaspoons Sunflower oil

1/2 cup organic white sugar

1/2 teaspoon Vitamin E

Directions:

1. Mix ingredients together in a large bowl.

2. Shelf Life: Store for up to a day in an air tight container.

Cinnamon Vanilla Body Scrub

Good for all types of skin. Regular use can lead to the reduction of wrinkles and fine lines as well.

Ingredients

1/2-3/4 cup raw sugar

1 cup brown sugar

2 tbsp raw honey

1/2 cup sea salt

1/4 cup coconut oil (liquefy if solid)

1/2 cup avocado oil

1 tsp cinnamon

1-2 tsp vanilla extract

1 tsp freshly grated nutmeg (optional)

5 drops nutmeg essential oil

5 drops cinnamon essential oil

Directions

1. Combine the salt and sugars.

2. Add avocado oil, vanilla extract, essential oils and spice(s).

3. Add to 2 half pint jars and enjoy!

Spicy Oat
Ingredients:

1/2 cup Oats

1/2 cup Brown rice

1/4 cup dried oregano

1/4 cup dried comfrey

1/2 cup Calendula

1/4 cup Myrrh

1/8 cup Anise seed

1 1/2 cups Clay

1 drop Lavender essential oil

1 drop Tea tree essential oil

Directions

1. Grind all ingredients except oils until powdery.

2. Add oils and then stir well then store in a jar.

3. To use: combine 1-2 teaspoon scrub and add a small amount of water.

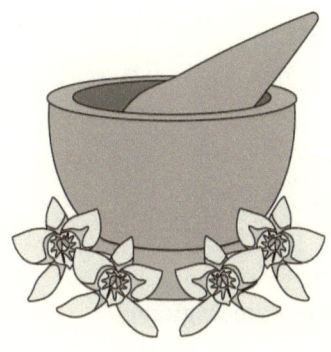

Lemon Milk Sugar

Ingredients:

1 cup Sugar

¼ cup Milk

2 tablespoons Olive oil

4 drops Lemon essential oil

Juice from one lemon

Directions:

1. Mix all ingredients well

2. Transfer the now gritty paste to an air tight container using a spoon.

3. Label, date and store in a cool place.

Oatmeal &Peels

A rejuvenating scrub for those who want to smell fresh all day long.

Ingredients:

1 cup dried Orange peels

1 cup Oatmeal

2 tablespoon Almonds, finely ground

1 teaspoon Sweet Orange essential oil

Directions:

1. Put ingredients in a food processor and mix thoroughly.

2. Take a little of this mix in your hand, add some warm water and make a paste.

3. Rub and massage onto your skin.

Peppermint Citrus

For dry, itchy skin

Ingredients:

1 cup Granulated white sugar

10-15 drops wild orange or grapefruit essential oil

10 drops Peppermint essential oil

1/4-1/3 cup olive, avocado or apricot oil both

2-4 tablespoon orange or grapefruit zest

2 tablespoon Vegetable glycerin

Directions:

1. Mix together sugar, zest, oil and vegetable glycerin.

2. Gently add essential oils until the desired scent is reached.

3. Store in a glass container.

Chamomile Petitgrain
Ingredients:

3 drops Chamomile essential oil

2 drops Petitgrain essential oil

1 cup Organic brown sugar

1/4 cup dried chamomile flowers

Directions:

1. Combine all the ingredients in a bowl.

2. Shelf Life: Store for up to a month in an air tight container.

Honey Herb Scrub
Good for irritated, sensitive or problem-prone skin.

Ingredients:

1/4 cup Honey

1 teaspoon dry sage

1 teaspoon dry thyme

1 teaspoon dry rosemary

1 cup Organic white sugar

Directions:

1. Combine ingredients and store.

2. Shelf Life: Store for up to a week in a sterilized glass jar.

Vanilla Patchouli

Ingredients:

1 cup Organic brown sugar

20 drops Vanilla fragrance oil

5 drops Patchouli essential oil

5 drops Ylang-ylang essential oil

Directions:

1. Mix ingredients together in a large bowl.

2. Shelf Life: Store for up to 6 months in an air tight container.

Peppermint-Citrus Salt Scrub

This body scrub smoothens, cleanses and stimulates the skin. It is useful for balancing oil production in normal, combination or oily and acne-prone skin.

Ingredients:

1 1/2 teaspoons Aloe Vera gel

1/2 cup sea salt

2 tablespoons other carrier oil of choice

2 drops rosemary essential oil

8 drops orange essential oil

5 drops peppermint essential oil

Directions:

1. Combine salt, Aloe Vera gel and oil in a ceramic bowl and stir.

2. Add the essential oils and stir again until well combined.

3. Usage: Take a warm shower; however, do not dry your body. Stand in the bathtub and rub the body scrub all over your skin with gentle circular motions.

4. Rinse off with water, dry your body and moisturize.

Caution: Do not use prior to sun exposure because the sweet orange essential oil may cause sunburn.

BATH RECIPES

(Bath salts, bath oils, bath bombs, bath teas, bubble baths, bath cookies, shower steamers, milk baths, face wash & body wash).

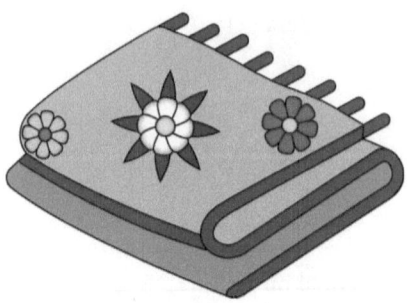

With the myriad of invigorating bath recipes available nowadays, it is unacceptable to have a plain and unexciting bath time! Containing essential oils, salts and other natural ingredients, these bath recipes are a healthy addition to your body. The inclusion of essential oils into your bath helps to hydrate and soften your skin as well as improve its tone and texture.

BATH SALTS

Bath salts contain anti-inflammatory properties and when combined with essential oils, you get to double the relief, rejuvenation and bliss that you'll enjoy. What's more, bath salts cleanse, detoxify, heal, and relieve pain. In addition, you get to soothe your nerves and bring down stress. You will really have a great energy boost whenever you use bath salts.

Recipes

Margarita Bath Salt
Ingredients:

1 cup Epsom salts

4-5 drops Green food coloring

10 drops Lime essential oil

Directions:

1. Combine all the ingredients: Epsom salts, essential oil and coloring and mix well.

2. Pour into in a small glass jar and seal. Leave it to set for several days.

3. Store in plastic bags or decorative jars.

4. Add bath salts into hot running or warm bath water. Soak liberally.

Aromatherapy Bath Salts
Ingredients:

2 1/2 cups Epsom salts

1 cup Baking Soda

1/2 cup Citric Acid

2 1/2 tsp Sweet Almond Oil

About 60 drops Ginger, peppermint and eucalyptus essential Oils

Directions

1. In a mixing bowl, combine all the dry ingredients until the entire clumps are broken.

2. Mix your essential oils and set aside. Add the sweet almond oil to your essential oils recipe.

3. Mix them all together and blend thoroughly. Package in a plastic bag.

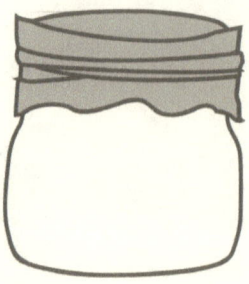

Seaside Bath Salt Soak

Ingredients:

¾ cups Epsom Salt

2 tsp Kelp Powder

1 tsp Powdered Grapefruit Peel

½ tsp spirulina Powder

1.4 oz Olive Oil

60 drops Rosemary Essential Oil

30 drops Juniper Essential Oil

20 drops Eucalyptus Essential Oil

Notes:

1. Grapefruit Peel powder, Kelp powder and Spirulina powder improves skin tone and promotes the synthesis of new collagen.

2. Besides Epsom salt, Sea Salt can also be use; just add a few scoops of it to warm running bath water.

Directions:

1. Mix all the ingredients in a small bowl.

2. Transfer to a glass jar and use within 60 days.

3. This recipe may cause the bath surface to become very slippery so be careful while using it.

Lemon Bath Salt

Ingredients:

1 cup Fine grain Sea Salt

1 cup Epsom Salt

3 tbsp Dendritic salt

1/2 tsp Lemon essential oil

1/2 tsp Vanilla Extract

5 drops Yellow 5 liquid dye

Directions:

1. Pour the fine grain Sea Salt and the Epsom Salt into a large stainless steel mixing bowl and then set aside.

2. In a separate but smaller mixing bowl, pour in the dendritic salt and add the vanilla extract and the lemon essential oil.

3. Mix very thoroughly and then add this mixture to the salts in the large stainless steel mixing bowl.

4. Mix thoroughly. Add yellow dye to the salt mixture and continue to mix well until the color is even throughout

5. Either use immediately or package well.

Oatmeal, Milk And Honey Salt Bath

Ingredients:

4 cups Powdered full cream/whole milk

1 cup Ground oats

1 cup Ground plain, raw almonds

1/2 cup Baking soda

1 cup Sea salt

2 cups Honey

4 drops Vanilla Essential oil

Notes:

Milk: Contains lactic acid which helps in breaking down and dissolving the proteins that hold together the dead skin cells. These dead skin cells must be removed in order for fresh new ones to resurface leading to a total youthful looking skin.

Honey : can absorb and retain moisture and this is why it is an essential ingredient in this recipe. It has natural antibacterial antifungal and antioxidant properties as well and this facilitates healing of different skin problems.

Oatmeal as well as baking soda is a wonderful exfoliant. It helps to soothe and heal rashes, sunburn and skin irritations. Grind oatmeal so that it will easily blend with the bath water and milk. It also draws toxin.

Directions:

1. Combine the sea salt, almond, oats, bathing soda and milk and then mix thoroughly.

2. Dissolve 4 cups of this powdered mixture in warm bath water (alternatively, you may pour the mix mixture into a cheesecloth bag, a clean

sock or coffee filter, tie it securely with a string and then soak in the bath water).

3. Add the honey and vanilla essential oil in the bath water and mix it thoroughly so it completely dissolves.

4. Soak your body in the bath for about 15 minutes. Rinse out the milk body under a warm shower.

5. Gently dry your skin with a clean towel.

Natural Grapefruit Bath Salts
Ingredients:

1 toe of a nylon stocking or cheesecloth

1 cup sea salt

2 drops pink food coloring

4 drops your favorite essential oil

Directions:

1. Place the salt in the toe of the stocking or on the cheesecloth.

2. Add the food coloring and essential oil. Fold up and tie with a string.

3. Add the bag to your bath water and wait for it to disperse slowly into the water. Soak for 20 or 30 minutes.

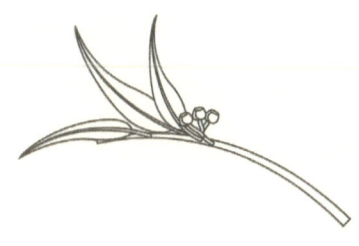

Ocean Bath Salts

Ingredients:

1 cup Epsom salt

2 tbsp Glycerin

1 cup Baking soda

4 drops Vanilla

4 drops Blue food coloring

3 drops Essential oil

Directions:

1. Combine dry ingredients and mix well. Add scents and color one at a time.

2. Continue to stir until thoroughly mixed. Break up any clumps.

3. Keep on mixing until a semi fine powder is formed. Add glycerin and mix well.

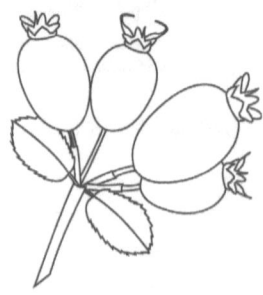

Rose-Scented Bath Salts

This bath salt recipe is great when you want to feel calm, happy and relaxed. Good for depression, daily stress, grief, menopause and PMS.

Ingredients:

3 cups Dead Sea salt

1/2 cup of baking soda

4 drops rose essential oil

1 drop ylang ylang essential oil

6 drops palmarosa essential oil

2 drops patchouli essential oil

4 drops rose geranium essential oil

10 drops of red food coloring

Directions:

1. In a bowl, add together salt and baking soda then stir together with a spoon.

2. Add essential oils and the food coloring. Stir to mix well.

3. Transfer the bath salts into a jar. Set aside to cure for 24 hours, at least.

4. Usage: 1 cup of the bath salt per bath. Pour into warm bath water and swirl it around to disperse.

5. Slide into the water and relax your body for 20 to 30 minutes.

BATH BOMB RECIPES

Bath times are pleasurable with bath bombs. Adults love their fragrance and look, while kids enjoy the fascination and fun that comes with making and using them. They make beautiful gifts too! These are besides it relaxing and cleansing advantages, of course. It is time to create your very own bath bomb with an essential oil that provides specific benefit that you desire.

<u>Recipes</u>

No- Citrus Acid Bath Bombs
For kids

Ingredients

2 cups baking soda

1 cup cream of tartar

1 tbsp olive oil

4-6 drops lavender essential oils

2- 3 sprays of water (spray bottle)

Ice cube trays

Directions

1. Combine all ingredients together in a bowl, except the water. Mix thoroughly.

2. Spray water and mix in thoroughly until it feels like wet sand.

3. Fill the silicon ice cube trays with this mixture, packing down firmly. Let it dry.

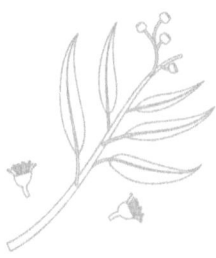

Scented Bath Bombs
Ingredients:

1 1/2 cups baking soda

1/2 cup citric acid

8 drops Essential oil of choice

1/2 tsp Sweet almond oil

2 drops Food coloring of choice

Directions

1. Combine all the ingredients and press into mould or muffin tin of choice.

2. Release from mould and wrap in plastic wraps and tie with a ribbon.

Fizzy Bath Bombs
Ingredients

1 1/2 cups baking soda

1/2 cup citric acid, powder

2 tsp sweet almond oil

6- 8 drops essential oil of choice

6 drops Food coloring

Directions:

1. Sift citric acid and baking soda together in a bowl.

2. Transfer half cup at a time to another dry bowl.

3. Mix together almond oil (1/2 teaspoon at a time), essential oil of choice & food coloring in a small bowl.

4. Pour the oil mix into the 1/2 cup base mix, mixing quickly before it begins to fizz! Combine color until evenly distributed.

5. Wipe sweet almond oil inside your molds. Let it set for at least 24 hours. Yields: 7

Cane Sugar Bath Bombs

Ingredients

½ cup powdered citric acid

¾ cup cornstarch

¼ cup cane sugar

1 cup baking soda

Essential oils

Food coloring

Directions

1. In a large bowl, incorporate dry ingredients (citric acid, cornstarch and baking soda) thoroughly. Add sugar and stir.

2. Add a little water using a spray bottle.

3. Once mixture becomes moldable in your hands, add food coloring and essential oil.

4. Press mixture into molds. Let the bombs dry and then store in an airtight container.

Dried Flower Bath Bombs

Ingredients

2 cups baking soda

1 cup citric acid

2 tablespoons coconut or argan oil

1 tbsp dried flower

10 drops essential oil of choice

Spray bottle with water (floral hydrosol may be added for extra scent)

Silicone molds

Directions

1. Mix the ingredients together in a bowl and then spray water into the mixture, mixing with hands.

2. (Mixture begins to bubble and becomes firm quickly) press them into molds.

3. Leave overnight to dry. Remove from mold.

4. Add 1 bomb to running bathwater and enjoy!

Peppermint Bath Bombs

Ingredients

1 cup baking soda

1/2 cup citric acid

10 drops peppermint essential

½ tbsp grape-seed oil

Spray bottle with water

Cosmetic mica powder for coloring (optional)

Silicone mold or muffin tin

Directions:

1. Combine the baking soda and citric acid in a bowl.

2. In another bowl, combine essential oil and carrier oil (grapeseed). Add it to the first mixture and stir well. For coloring, add mica powder, if desired.

3. Use a spray water bottle to mist the surface until a bit damp.

4. Pack into molds covered with paper towel. (For small heart shapes, use silicone and for larger, use a muffin tin). Place on baking sheet. Unmold and let dry overnight.

Minty Eucalyptus Bath Bombs

Ingredients:

½ cup citric acid

1 cup baking soda

2 tbsp jojoba oil

5 drops lemon essential oil

5 drops peppermint essential oil

5 drops eucalyptus essential oil

1 tbsp. witch hazel

Directions:

1. Combine citric acid and baking soda in a mixing bowl.

2. Drizzle in jojoba oil and essential oils. Mix thoroughly until smooth.

3. Drizzle in witch hazel slowly, continuously stirring so the ingredients do not fizz.

4. Once mixture is moist enough to clump together, press firmly into molds.

5. Let bombs dry for 3 to 4 hours then remove from the molds.

6. Recipe makes 6-10 bath bombs.

Goat's Milk Bath Bombs

Ingredients

1 ¼ cups baking soda

1/2 cup citric acid

1/4 cup powdered goat's milk

2 tsp apricot kernel oil

1/2 tbsp water

10-15 drops musk essential oil

Directions

1. Combine all the dry ingredients in a bowl, stirring until well mixed.

2. Drizzle in the apricot kernel oil, stirring until mixture is moistened. Add essential oil and stir until well mixed. Add water.

3. Pack firmly into mold and leave to dry. Use 1 bomb per bath.

Rooibos Detox Bombs

Ingredients

2 tsp organic Rooibos leaves

1 tbsp citric acid

2 tbsp baking soda

2 tbsp cornflower

1-2 tsp pure olive oil

Chamomile essential oil

Turmeric to color

Directions

1. Sieve dry ingredients in a bowl, mixing well. Add Rooibos leaves, fragrance oil and color

2. Blend well until thoroughly blended.

3. Spritz lightly with witch hazel or water, mixing in well.

4. The mixture should stay together if squeezed, otherwise mist/ spritz lightly with witch hazel or water and mix again. Repeat until it holds together.

5. Lightly squash some mist into your mold halves (dome top with extra mixture).

6. Push the two halves quickly together and firmly squeeze. To ensure a good shape, line edges of mold. Remove one half of mold immediately and tip out gently to place on wax paper.

7. Leave to harden for at least 24 hours. Package in an airtight container or wrap in cellophane and tie with a bow.

8. Usage: drop bomb in warm bath and fizz away.

Dried Flower Bath Bombs

Ingredients

2 cups baking soda

1 cup citric acid

2 tablespoons coconut or argan oil

1 tbsp dried flower

10 drops essential oil of choice

Spray bottle with water (floral hydrosol may be added for extra scent)

Silicone molds

Directions

1. Mix the ingredients together in a bowl and then spray water into the mixture, mixing with hands.

2. (Mixture begins to bubble and becomes firm quickly) press them into molds.

3. Leave overnight to dry. Remove from mold.

4. Add 1 bomb to running bathwater and enjoy!

Lavender & Oatmeal Bath Bombs
Ingredients

1/4 cup quick oats

1/2 cup citric acid

1 cup baking soda

1/8 tsp Rose Geranium essential oil

1/4 tsp Lavender essential oil

Flower petals (Rose petals &Lavender buds)

Witch Hazel - in a spray bottle

Note: Lavender oil as a bomb bath ingredient is a natural de-stressor. Lavender has been used for thousands of years as a mild sedative which help to reduce stress, anxiety and induce restful sleep.

Directions:

1. Mix the baking soda and citric acid together in a large bowl, mixing thoroughly and breaking up any clumps with your fingers.

2. Once mixture is smooth, add the quick oats and mix well. Drizzle essential oils on top and mix in thoroughly.

3. Spray mixture with witch hazel until a slightly damp consistency is attained. (Spray 3 squirts at a time, mix, spray again and mix until mixture holds in your hand when squeezed).

4. Place dried flower petals at bottom of one half of bomb mold. Leave for several hours to harden.

5. Store in tin foil to prevent moisture. This recipe makes 3medium round bath fizzies (6cm / 2.25" diameter) and 1 mini.

BATH OILS

A scented warm bath helps your body to recover from the wear and tear of the day. They give you an opportunity to relax and eliminate stress. Now when essential oil is added to the bath it will nourish your body at deeper levels while the carrier oils will provide hydration and nourishment for your skin.

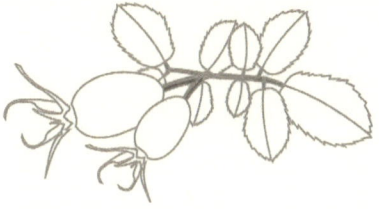

Recipes

Simple Aromatherapy Bath Oil

Ingredients:

15-30 drops Essential oil of choice

1 1/2 oz Olive oil

1 oz Canola oil

1 oz Sesame oil

3 oz Almond oil

1/2 oz Wheat germ oil

Directions:

1. Fill a small- mouth jar with all the carrier oils and leave eave 1 /8 inch of space at the top.

2. Next, gradually add the essential oil then use a tight lid to cap the jar and shake thoroughly

3. Use 2 teaspoons of oil per bath.

Blissful Oil Bath

Ingredients:

10 drops Sandalwood

5 drops Jasmine

5 drops Rose

5 drops Bergamot

4tbsp Jojoba, Castor, Almond or simple Sunflower base oil

Directions:

1. Pour base oil into a glass jar or bottle. Add essential oil. Cover and shake thoroughly.

2. Store in a dark place and leave for 2weeks to mature.

3. Once matured, add 1 tablespoon of the scented oil to the bath. Swish to disburse.

4. Enjoy your blissful oil bath and remain happy.

Muscle Relaxing Bath Oil Blend

Ingredients

2 ounces jojoba or almond oil

7 drops Rosemary essential oil

8 drops Lavender essential oil

5 drops Eucalyptus essential oil

Directions:

1. Combine all ingredients and pour into tub of warm water as tub fills.

2. Soak in the tub for 15 minutes

Sensuous Oil Bath
Ingredients:

20 drops Jasmine essential oil

8 drops Orange essential oil

4tbs jojoba, Castor, Almond or simple Sunflower base oils

Directions:

1. Pour base oil into a glass jar or bottle. Add essential oil. Cover and shake thoroughly.

2. Store in a dark place and leave for 2weeks to mature.

3. Once matured, add 1 tablespoon of the scented oil to the bath. Swish to disburse.

4. Enjoy your sensual oil bath.

Revitalizing Oil Bath
Ingredients:

12 drops Geranium essential oil

6 drops Sandalwood essential oil

6 drops Lemon essential oil

2 drops Clary Sage essential oil

4tbsp Jojoba, Castor, Almond or simple Sunflower base oils

Directions:

1. Pour base oil into a glass jar or bottle. Add essential oil. Cover and shake thoroughly.

2. Store in a dark place and leave for 2weeks to mature.

3. Once matured, add 1 tablespoon of the scented oil to the bath. Swish to disburse.

4. Enjoy your revitalizing oil bath to relive stress and depression

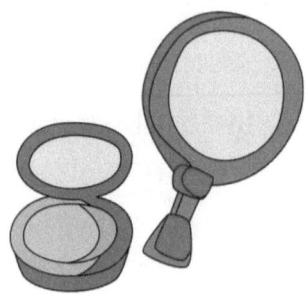

Relaxing Oil Bath
Ingredients:

12 drops Sandalwood essential oil

8 drops Orange essential oil

4 drops Rose essential oil

2 drops Pine essential oil

2 drops Lemon essential oil

4tbsp of Jojoba, Castor, Almond or simple Sunflower base oils

Directions

1. Pour base oil into a glass jar or bottle. Add essential oil. Cover and shake thoroughly.

2. Store in a dark place and leave for 2weeks to mature.

3. Once matured, add 1 tablespoon of the scented oil to the bath. Swish to disburse.

4. Enjoy your relaxing oil bath to relive stress and depression.

Shampoo Bath Oil
Ingredients:

10 drops Essential oil of choice

4 tbsp Mild baby shampoo

125ml Almond or Sunflower oil

 Note:

Baby shampoo is an effective carrier that helps to quickly and evenly disburse your oils.

Directions:

1. Pour base oil into a glass jar. Add the shampoo and shake well.

2. Add essential oil, shake well. Leave for 2 weeks to mature but keep way from daylight.

3. Once matured, add 2 tablespoons per bath and swish to disperse.Enjoy your bath.

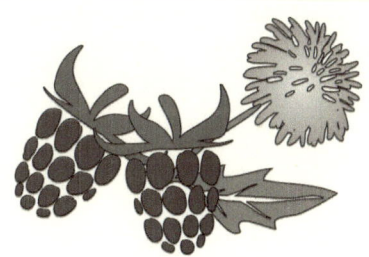

Lavender Soothing Bath Oil

This pain-relieving, relaxing and sleep-inducing blend will help you unwind. It is also good for insomnia, stress, colds and flu.

Ingredients:

10 drops lavender essential oil

1 drop cedarwood essential oil

5 drops marjoram essential oil

5 drops frankincense essential oil

4 ounces jojoba or sweet almond oil (or other carrier oil of your choice)

Directions:

1. Combine all ingredients in a dark glass bottle.

2. Store in a cool and dark place.

3. To use, pour a tablespoon of it into a warm bath water and swirl it around to disperse.

4. Slide into the water and relax for 20- 30 minutes.

Soothing Aromatherapy Bath Oil

Feel your stress melting away with this yummy bath blend with a deep woodsy scent that is also good for men.

Ingredients:

12 drops lavender essential oil

2 drops cedarwood essential oil

30 drops of sandalwood essential oil

4 ounces jojoba or sweet almond oil

Directions:

1. Combine all ingredients in a dark glass bottle.

2. Store in a cool and dark place.

3. To use, pour a tablespoon of it into a warm bath water and swirl it around to disperse.

4. Slide into the water and relax for 20- 30 minutes.

Alcohol Bath Oil

Ingredients:

100ml Castor Oil

4 tbsp Vodka or brandy

10 drops Essential oils of choice

Note: Spirits help in the quick and even distribution of the oil.

Directions:

1. Pour the castor oil into a glass jar. Add the spirit and shake well

2. Add essential oil, shake thoroughly.

3. Leave for 2 weeks to mature but keep way from daylight.

4. Once matured, add 2 tablespoons per bath and swish to disperse. Enjoy your bath.

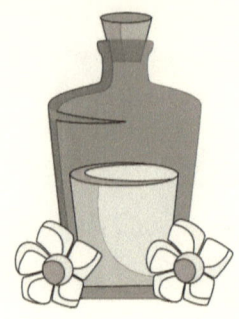

10 Top Singular Bath Oil Recipes:

These are my 10 best singular bath oils for different purposes.

Treatment	Essential oil	Quantity
Depression	Bergamot oil	5 drops
Stress or fatigue	Jasmine	8 drops
Soothing and relaxing	Lavender	10 drops
Insomnia or itchy skin	Chamomile	7 drops
Sensual and mellowing a great aphrodisiac	Sandalwood	8 drops
Happiness and romantic pleasure	Rose	10 drops
Relaxing, uplifting and energizing	Geranium	10 drops
hypnotic with antidepressant properties	Neroli	7 drops
energizing and invigorating	Patchouli	5 drops
sedative and mood sweetening	Frankincense	8 drops

BUBBLE BATH RECIPES

Bath time is fun with bubble baths. With essential oils, you can try various scents and still benefit from their therapeutic properties.

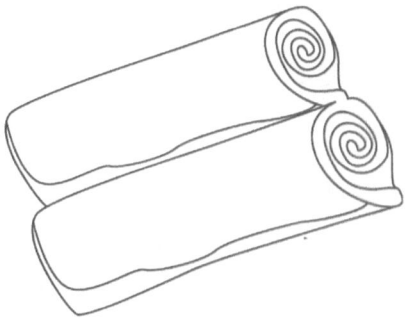

Recipes

Citrus Sunshine Bubble Bath

Ingredients:

1/2 tablespoon white sugar

1 1/2 cups of liquid castile soap

2 tablespoons vegetable glycerin

1 drop rose geranium essential oil or ylang ylang

4 drops orange essential oil

5 drops bergamot essential oil

5 drops food coloring of choice

Directions:

1. Gently stir together all ingredients in a large glass bowl.

2. Remove the bubble bath to a clean dark glass jar. Leave for at least 24 hours to cure. Store in a cool, dark place.

3. Usage: 1/4 cup bubble bath per bath. Pour into warm bath water then swirl around to disperse.

4. Enter into the water and relax your body for 20 to 30 minutes.

Caution: orange and bergamot may cause sunburn therefore, do not use prior to sun exposure.

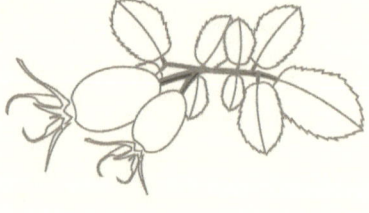

Lavender Uplifting Bubble Bath
Ingredients:

1 drop chamomile essential oil

1/2 tablespoon white sugar

2 tablespoons vegetable glycerin

5 drops lavender essential oil

4 drops lemon essential oil

5 drops food coloring of choice

1 1/2 cups of liquid castile soap

Directions:

1. Gently stir together all ingredients in a large glass bowl.

2. Remove the bubble bath to a clean dark glass jar. Leave for at least 24 hours to cure. Store in a cool, dark place.

3. <u>Usage:</u> 1/4 cup bubble bath per bath. Pour into warm bath water then swirl around to disperse.

4. Enter into the water and relax your body for 20 to 30 minutes.

Silky And Spicy Bubble Bath

Ingredients:

5 drops lavender essential oil

1 1/2 cups of liquid castile soap

2 tablespoons vegetable glycerin

4 drops sandalwood essential oil

1 drop clove essential oil

1/2 tablespoon white sugar

5 drops food coloring of choice

Directions:

1. Gently stir together all ingredients in a large glass bowl.

2. Remove the bubble bath to a clean dark glass jar. Leave for at least 24 hours to cure. Store in a cool, dark place.

3. <u>Usage:</u> 1/4 cup bubble bath per bath. Pour into warm bath water then swirl around to disperse.

4. Enter into the water and relax your body for 20 to 30 minutes.

Caution: Do not use clove essential oil if you have sensitive skin.

Rose Absolute Bubble Bath

Ingredients:

1 1/2 cups of liquid castile soap

1/2 tablespoon white sugar

2 tablespoons vegetable glycerin

3 drops rose absolute essential oil

2 drops palmarosa essential oil

1 drop rose geranium essential oil

5 drops food coloring of choice

Directions:

1. Gently stir together all ingredients in a large glass bowl.

2. Remove the bubble bath to a clean dark glass jar. Leave for at least 24 hours to cure. Store in a cool, dark place.

3. Usage: 1/4 cup bubble bath per bath. Pour into warm bath water then swirl around to disperse.

4. Enter into the water and relax your body for 20 to 30 minutes.

Sweet Vanilla Bubble Bath

Ingredients:

6 drops vanilla absolute essential oil

1 1/2 cups of liquid castile soap

2 tablespoons vegetable glycerin

1/2 tablespoon white sugar

5 drops food coloring of choice

Directions:

1. Gently stir together all ingredients in a large glass bowl.

2. Remove the bubble bath to a clean dark glass jar. Leave for at least 24 hours to cure. Store in a cool, dark place.

3. <u>Usage:</u> 1/4 cup bubble bath per bath. Pour into warm bath water then swirl around to disperse.

4. Enter into the water and relax your body for 20 to 30 minutes.

MILK BATH RECIPES

Milk bath recipes are ideal for people who wish to rejuvenate their skin's vitality. When your skin is feeling dry, all you need to do is soak for a few minutes in any of the soothing preparations below. The milk content in the recipe will soften the skin and remove the layer of dead cells that clog the surface. To get more nourishment, use milk with higher fat content. Additionally, the essential oils in each recipe provide extra benefits.

Recipes

Plain Milk Bath

Ingredients:

2 cups powdered milk, non-fat

1 cup Cornstarch

5 drops Essential oil

Directions:

1. Mix ingredients well.

2. Boil water and once hot add 1/2 cup of mixture to it.

3. Enjoy a refreshing bath.

Skin Softening Milk Bath

Ingredients

3 tablespoons Epsom salt

1 cup buttermilk

3 drops lavender essential oil

½ tablespoon olive oil

Directions:

1. Combine all ingredients and pour into tub of warm water as tub fills.

2. Soak in the tub for 15-20 minutes and then wash off afterwards.

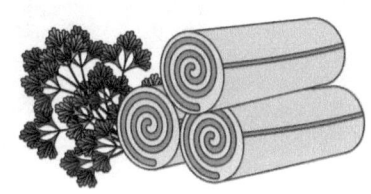

Sweet Vanilla Milk Bath

Ingredients:

2 cups of whole powdered milk

12 drops of vanilla absolute essential oil

1/4 cup baking soda

1/2 cup cornstarch

Directions:

1. Add together powdered milk, cornstarch and baking soda in a dark glass jar.

2. Cover and shake to mix thoroughly.

3. Add the essential oil, cover the jar and shake to combine.

4. Set aside to cure for 24 hours, at least

5. <u>Usage:</u> Pour 1- 2 cups of the milk bath directly under running bath water. Swirl with your hands to disperse.

6. Slide into the water and relax for 20 to 30 minutes.

7. Apply body oil or a hydrating lotion to finish off.

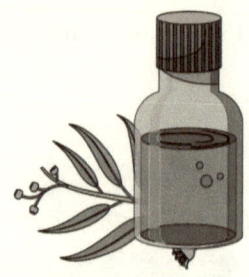

Meadow Milk Bath
Ingredients:

4 oz powdered milk, finely sifted

2 oz Citric Acid

2 oz Corn starch

30 drops Grapefruit Seed Oil

60 drops Jasmine essential oil

Directions

1. Blend the corn starch and powdered milk and then sift.

2. Mix the grapefruit seed oil and Jasmine in Citric Acid, ensuring the oils are well blended in the Citric Acid

3. Add the Citric Acid blend to the milk/corn starch blend. Use 3 tablespoons to each bath.

Lavender Milk Bath
Ingredients:

1 cup powdered milk

2-3 drops Lavender essential oil

Directions:

1. Mix ingredients together

2. Add to bath.

Spicy And Silky Milk Bath
Ingredients:

2 cups of whole powdered milk

9 drops sandalwood essential oil

1/4 cup baking soda

10 drops lavender essential oil

1/2 cup cornstarch

1 drop clove essential oil

Directions:

1. Add together powdered milk, cornstarch and baking soda in a dark glass jar.

2. Cover and shake to mix thoroughly.

3. Add the essential oil, cover the jar and shake to combine.

4. Set aside to cure for 24 hours, at least

5. Usage: Pour 1- 2 cups of the milk bath directly under running bath water. Swirl with your hands to disperse.

6. Slide into the water and relax for 20 to 30 minutes.

7. Apply body oil or a hydrating lotion to finish off.

Caution: Leave out clove if you have sensitive skin.

Rose Absolute Milk Bath

Ingredients:

2 cups of whole powdered milk

1 drop rose geranium essential oil

1/4 cup baking soda

6 drops rose absolute essential oil

1/2 cup cornstarch

3 drops palmarosa essential oil

Directions:

1. Add together powdered milk, cornstarch and baking soda in a dark glass jar.

2. Cover and shake to mix thoroughly.

3. Add the essential oil, cover the jar and shake to combine.

4. Set aside to cure for 24 hours, at least

5. Usage: Pour 1- 2 cups of the milk bath directly under running bath water. Swirl with your hands to disperse.

6. Slide into the water and relax for 20 to 30 minutes.

7. Apply body oil or a hydrating lotion to finish off.

BATH TEAS & OTHER RECIPES

Essential oil bath tea recipes are great when you want to treat your body to some tender loving care. Essential oils' fragrance and healing ability work together with other natural ingredients to nourish your skin, relax your muscles, calm nerves and elevate your mood.

Recipes

Relaxing Bath Tea

Ingredients:

4 oz. Lavender flowers

4 oz. Chamomile flowers

2 oz Calendula petals

20 drops Bulgarian Lavender EO

Directions

1. Combine ingredients and package.

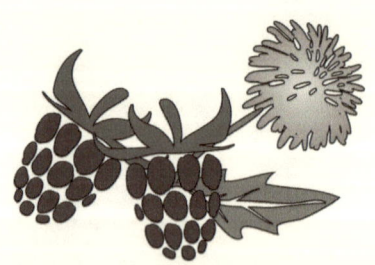

Green Herbal Bath Tea

A bath tea recipe that is filled with nourishing herbs to soothe your nerves and soften your skin.

Ingredients:

1/2 cup rose petals

1/2 cup lavender flowers

1/4 cup green tea leaves (jasmine or rose flavored tea)

3 drops lavender essential oil

1 drop rose geranium essential oil

3 drops rose or palmarosa essential oil

Directions:

1. In a dark glass jar, add together the rose petals, tea leaves and lavender flowers.

2. Add the essential oils, stirring together gently with a spoon.

3. Combine all together in a dark glass jar.

4. Cover the jar and leave it to cure for at least 24 hours.

5. Usage: Put 2-3 spoonfuls in a small organza drawstring or muslin bag. Cheesecloth tied with a string can also be used.

6. In a kettle, bring water to a boil then steep the herbal bath tea bag for 10 minutes.

7. Pour the herbal tea water into your prepared bath water then throw in the bag.

8. Slide into the water and relax for 20- 30 minutes.

9. Do not rinse your body. Simply pat dry with a towel then apply a natural body lotion.

Oatmeal Herbal Bath Tea

This nourishing oatmeal bath recipe works on dry and problematic skin to soothe and moisturize it. It also relieves irritation, itchiness and inflammation. Good for psoriasis, eczema and acne.

Ingredients:

2 cups of rolled oats

4 drops chamomile essential oil

3 drops palmarosa essential oil

4 drops of lavender essential oil

3 tablespoons chamomile flowers

3 tablespoons lavender flowers

Directions:

1. Put the oats in a blender and grind until you have a coarse powder.

2. Combine the ground oats with lavender and chamomile flowers in a large bowl.

3. Add the essential oils, stirring together gently with a spoon. Combine all together in a dark glass jar.

4. Cover the jar and leave it to cure for at least 24 hours.

5. Usage: Put 2-3 spoonfuls in a small organza drawstring or muslin bag. Cheesecloth tied with a string can also be used.

6. In a kettle, bring water to a boil then steep the herbal bath tea bag for 10 minutes.

7. Pour the herbal tea water into your prepared bath water then throw in the bag.

8. Slide into the water and relax for 20- 30 minutes.

9. Do not rinse your body. Simply pat dry with a towel then apply a natural body lotion.

SHOWER STEAMER RECIPES

If you like having fun in the bathroom, these are lovely products you should make. They make wonderful gifts too! They are fizzy little gems that everyone will love.

<u>Recipes</u>

Revitalizing Shower Steamer

Ingredients:

2 cups baking soda

1 cup citric acid

1 spray bottle of witch hazel

30 drops peppermint essential oil

30 drops lemon essential oil

5 drops basil or geranium essential oil

Directions:

1. Sift the baking soda and citric acid with a fine sieve,, pressing to remove lumps. Stir well the mixture.

2. Add the essential oils and stir again to combine.

3. Spray some witch hazel on the mixture, stirring vigorously with a fork or even your fingers.

4. Keep spraying and stirring until the mixture binds well when squeezed but it shouldn't be wet. It is ready when it holds its shape after being squeezed together with your hands.

5. Now, press your shower steamer tightly and firmly into molds (like candy molds or silicone muffin tins). Press down well into the mold so it is thoroughly packed.

6. Set aside for 1 hour then flip over each mold and tap out the shower steamers gently onto a flat surface.

7. Cover them loosely with a piece of plastic wrap then set aside for several hours to fully dry.

8. Wrap up the dry shower steamers with plastic wrap or parchment paper and store in an air-tight container.

9. To use, place the shower steamer on the floor while taking a shower, and let it steam away. A burst of scent will be released each time the spray hits it.

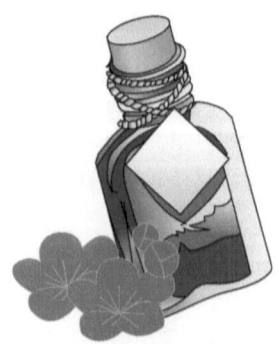

Anti-Stuffiness Shower Steamer

This recipe is good for colds and congestion.

Ingredients:

2 cups baking soda

1 cup citric acid

1 spray bottle of witch hazel

25 drops eucalyptus essential oil

30 drops peppermint essential oil

10 drops tea tree essential oil

Directions:

1. Sift the baking soda and citric acid with a fine sieve,, pressing to remove lumps. Stir well the mixture.

2. Add the essential oils and stir again to combine.

3. Spray some witch hazel on the mixture, stirring vigorously with a fork or even your fingers.

4. Keep spraying and stirring until the mixture binds well when squeezed but it shouldn't be wet. It is ready when it holds its shape after being squeezed together with your hands.

5. Now, press your shower steamer tightly and firmly into molds (like candy molds or silicone muffin tins). Press down well into the mold so it is thoroughly packed.

6. Set aside for 1 hour then flip over each mold and tap out the shower steamers gently onto a flat surface.

7. Cover them loosely with a piece of plastic wrap then set aside for several hours to fully dry.

8. Wrap up the dry shower steamers with plastic wrap or parchment paper and store in an air-tight container.

9. To use, place the shower steamer on the floor while taking a shower, and let it steam away. A burst of scent will be released each time the spray hits it.

After Workout Shower Steamer
Ingredients:

2 cups baking soda

1 cup citric acid

1 spray bottle of witch hazel

25 drops lavender essential oil

30 drops grapefruit essential oil

10 drops peppermint essential oil

Directions:

1. Sift the baking soda and citric acid with a fine sieve,, pressing to remove lumps. Stir well the mixture.

2. Add the essential oils and stir again to combine.

3. Spray some witch hazel on the mixture, stirring vigorously with a fork or even your fingers.

4. Keep spraying and stirring until the mixture binds well when squeezed but it shouldn't be wet. It is ready when it holds its shape after being squeezed together with your hands.

5. Now, press your shower steamer tightly and firmly into molds (like candy molds or silicone muffin tins). Press down well into the mold so it is thoroughly packed.

6. Set aside for 1 hour then flip over each mold and tap out the shower steamers gently onto a flat surface.

7. Cover them loosely with a piece of plastic wrap then set aside for several hours to fully dry.

8. Wrap up the dry shower steamers with plastic wrap or parchment paper and store in an air-tight container.

9. To use, place the shower steamer on the floor while taking a shower, and let it steam away. A burst of scent will be released each time the spray hits it.

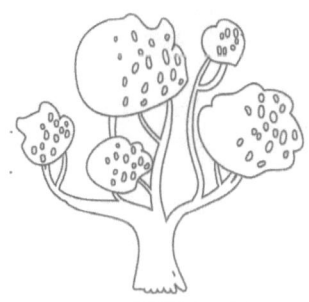

Elevating Shower Steamer

Use this when you are cranky or depressed.

Ingredients:

2 cups baking soda

1 cup citric acid

1 spray bottle of witch hazel

30 drops bergamot, grapefruit or lemon essential oil

3 drops rosemary essential oil

2 drops geranium essential oil

5 drops frankincense essential oil

25 drops lavender essential oil

Directions:

1. Sift the baking soda and citric acid with a fine sieve,, pressing to remove lumps. Stir well the mixture.

2. Add the essential oils and stir again to combine.

3. Spray some witch hazel on the mixture, stirring vigorously with a fork or even your fingers.

4. Keep spraying and stirring until the mixture binds well when squeezed but it shouldn't be wet. It is ready when it holds its shape after being squeezed together with your hands.

5. Now, press your shower steamer tightly and firmly into molds (like candy molds or silicone muffin tins). Press down well into the mold so it is thoroughly packed.

6. Set aside for 1 hour then flip over each mold and tap out the shower steamers gently onto a flat surface.

7. Cover them loosely with a piece of plastic wrap then set aside for several hours to fully dry.

8. Wrap up the dry shower steamers with plastic wrap or parchment paper and store in an air-tight container.

9. To use, place the shower steamer on the floor while taking a shower, and let it steam away. A burst of scent will be released each time the spray hits it.

Relaxing Shower Steamer

Beat insomnia with this recipe and have a restful night.

Ingredients:

1 cup citric acid

1 spray bottle of witch hazel

2 cups baking soda

30 drops lavender essential oil

15 drops sandalwood essential oil

15 drops frankincense essential oil

3 drops vetiver essential oil

2 drops geranium essential oil

Directions:

1. Sift the baking soda and citric acid with a fine sieve,, pressing to remove lumps. Stir well the mixture.

2. Add the essential oils and stir again to combine.

3. Spray some witch hazel on the mixture, stirring vigorously with a fork or even your fingers.

4. Keep spraying and stirring until the mixture binds well when squeezed but it shouldn't be wet. It is ready when it holds its shape after being squeezed together with your hands.

5. Now, press your shower steamer tightly and firmly into molds (like candy molds or silicone muffin tins). Press down well into the mold so it is thoroughly packed.

6. Set aside for 1 hour then flip over each mold and tap out the shower steamers gently onto a flat surface.

7. Cover them loosely with a piece of plastic wrap then set aside for several hours to fully dry.

8. Wrap up the dry shower steamers with plastic wrap or parchment paper and store in an air-tight container.

9. To use, place the shower steamer on the floor while taking a shower, and let it steam away. A burst of scent will be released each time the spray hits it.

Spicy Shower Steamer

Ingredients:

1 spray bottle of witch hazel

1 cup citric acid

2 cups baking soda

25 drops patchouli essential oil

5 drops clove essential oil

35 drops lavender essential oil

Directions:

1. Sift the baking soda and citric acid with a fine sieve,, pressing to remove lumps. Stir well the mixture.

2. Add the essential oils and stir again to combine.

3. Spray some witch hazel on the mixture, stirring vigorously with a fork or even your fingers.

4. Keep spraying and stirring until the mixture binds well when squeezed but it shouldn't be wet. It is ready when it holds its shape after being squeezed together with your hands.

5. Now, press your shower steamer tightly and firmly into molds (like candy molds or silicone muffin tins). Press down well into the mold so it is thoroughly packed.

6. Set aside for 1 hour then flip over each mold and tap out the shower steamers gently onto a flat surface.

7. Cover them loosely with a piece of plastic wrap then set aside for several hours to fully dry.

8. Wrap up the dry shower steamers with plastic wrap or parchment paper and store in an air-tight container.

9. To use, place the shower steamer on the floor while taking a shower, and let it steam away. A burst of scent will be released each time the spray hits it.

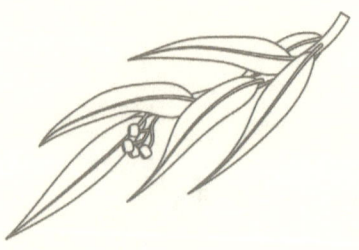

Other Bath Recipes

Easy Homemade Shower Gel

Enjoy the beautiful scent while showering! With this blend, you will think you died and went to heaven with this blend!

Ingredients

2/3 cup castile soap

1 tsp vitamin E oil

2 Tbsp raw honey

1 tsp jojoba oil

10 drops Ylang Ylang essential oil

5 drops spruce essential oil

2 tsp vegetable glycerin

Directions

1. Whisk all ingredients to combine well.

2. Fill an 8 oz. mason jar and top with soap pump lid.

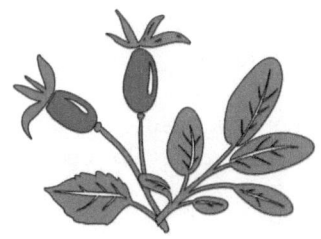

Lavender & Chamomile Bath Melts

Ingredients:

¼ cup organic Shea butter

¼ cup organic cocoa butter

2 drops lavender essential oil

1 tsp dried lavender flowers

1 tsp organic chamomile tea

Directions:

1. Thinly grate the cocoa butter and pour in a glass bowl. Add the Shea butter as well.

2. Place your glass bowl on a pan of hot water, stir until it melts then remove from heat.

3. Sprinkle organic chamomile tea into the mix. Add the dried lavender and stir thoroughly.

4. Pour the molten mix carefully into silicone moulds (ice cube trays can also be used). Add the lavender essential oil to the moulds.

5. Refrigerate your melts for an hour to harden. Once hardened, pop the melts from their mould and store in a fine glass jar.

6. How To Use:

1. Pop a bath melt in a warm bath and then wait till it dissolves.

2. The cocoa butter may make your bath a little slippery so you've got to be careful.

3. However, you can put your bath melt in a muslin cloth bag if you do not want the chamomile and lavender flowers to cover your bath.

FACIAL STEAMS RECIPES
(Facial Saunas)

Facial steams are a wonderful way to have facial saunas in your home and enjoy the opportunity of cleansing your face and revitalizing your skin once a week. They work for acne-prone and oily skin. Face steams open up pores and your skin can effortlessly get rid of excess oil, deep-down dirt and grime. Also, you can have a facial sauna then use a facial mask.

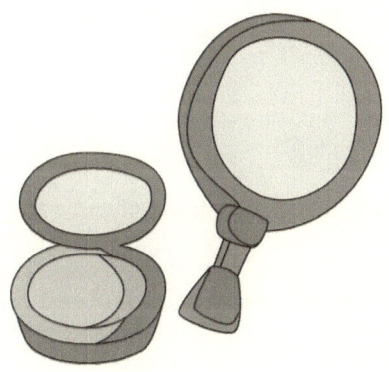

Recipes

Facial Steam For Normal And Combination Skin
A sweetly scented steam that will cleanse, open up and soothe your skin.

Ingredients:

2 tablespoons dried calendula

2 tablespoons dried chamomile

2 tablespoons dried rose petals

2 tablespoons of dried lavender flowers

1 drop rose geranium essential oil

69

2 drops palmarosa essential oil

1 drop chamomile essential oil

5 drops lavender essential oil

1 drop ylang ylang essential oil

Directions:

1. In a dark glass jar, combine the dried herbs and flowers.

2. Add the essential oils and shake thoroughly.

3. Set aside to cure for 24 hours, at least.

4. Usage: In a large pot, throw a handful of the mixture, add 1 to 2 quarts of water and bring to a boil.

5. Remove from heat and let it steep, covered for 5 minutes.

6. Remove the lid, place the pot on a low table then use a towel to make a tent on your head together with the pot of steaming herbs and oils.

7. Remain this tent for 5-10 minutes, coming out for air as necessary. Do not let your face burn.

Facial Steam For Mature, Dry And Sensitive Skin

Create a steam that soothes dry or irritated skin with the combination of ingredients in this recipe.

Ingredients:

2 tablespoons dried elder flower

2 tablespoons dried chamomile

2 tablespoons dried rose petals

1 drop chamomile essential oil

2 drops helichrysum essential oil

1 drop rose essential oil

5 drops frankincense essential oil

2 drops sandalwood essential oil

Directions:

1. In a dark glass jar, combine the dried herbs and flowers.

2. Add the essential oils and shake thoroughly.

3. Set aside to cure for 24 hours, at least.

4. Usage: In a large pot, throw a handful of the mixture, add 1 to 2 quarts of water and bring to a boil.

5. Remove from heat and let it steep, covered for 5 minutes.

6. Remove the lid, place the pot on a low table then use a towel to make a tent on your head together with the pot of steaming herbs and oils.

7. Remain this tent for 5-10 minutes, coming out for air as necessary. Do not let your face burn.

Facial Steam For Acne And Oily Skin

This face steam provides cleaning, healing and refreshing benefits that are vital for oily and acne-prone skin.

Ingredients:

2 tablespoons dried peppermint leaves

1/4 cup dried parsley leaves

1/4 cup dried lavender flowers

5 drops lemon or bergamot essential oil

1/4 cup dried rosemary leaves

10 drops lavender essential oil

Directions:

1. In a dark glass jar, combine the dried herbs and flowers.

2. Add the essential oils and shake thoroughly.

3. Set aside to cure for 24 hours, at least.

4. <u>Usage:</u> In a large pot, throw a handful of the mixture, add 1 to 2 quarts of water and bring to a boil.

5. Remove from heat and let it steep, covered for 5 minutes.

6. Remove the lid, place the pot on a low table then use a towel to make a tent on your head together with the pot of steaming herbs and oils.

7. Remain this tent for 5-10 minutes, coming out for air as necessary. Do not let your face burn.

FACIAL MASKS RECIPES

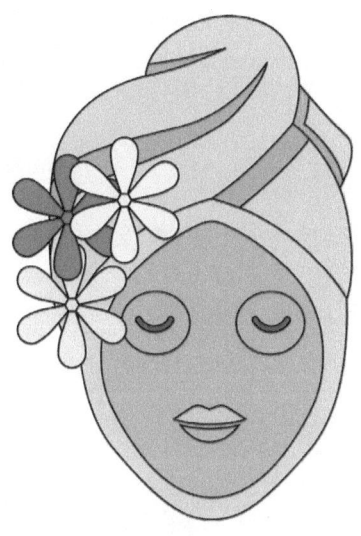

Recipes

Essential Oil Blackhead Removal Mask

Ingredients:

1 tablespoon gelatin

1 drop frankincense essential oil

1 drop peppermint essential oil

½ teaspoon turmeric

Directions:

1. Add 1/8 cup of water to a pan and heat.

2. Place the warm water in a small bowl and add the peppermint essential oil. Stir and add the gelatin and stir again.

3. Next, add the frankincense. Stir and add the turmeric, stirring to blend well.

4. Apply to the nose and cheek area or entire face area. Let it dry then peel off gently and rinse with warm water.

Face Mask For Normal Skin

Yummy and super-refreshing, this homemade face with drops of essential oil mask hydrates and cleanses the skin. Use it weekly to help prevent and possibly reduce visible signs of aging.

Ingredients:

1/4 teaspoon jojoba oil

1 tablespoon cosmetic clay

1/2 teaspoon honey

1 teaspoon yogurt or milk

1 drop lavender essential oil

1 drop rose geranium essential oil

Directions:

1. Whisk together honey, jojoba oil, yogurt and essential oils in a small bowl.

2. Stir in the clay, gradually until a paste of desired consistency is attained. Do not make it too thick.

3. Cleanse your face and neck area.

4. Apply the mask to your face and neck, while still damp, taking care to avoid eyes and mouth. Throw away any remainder.

5. Let it stay for 15 to 20 minutes.

6. Wash off with a wet and warm washcloth then apply a toner and moisturizer.

Face Mask For Dry And Mature Skin

With easy-to-find and inexpensive items, this is a wonderful moisturizing and nourishing face mask for your skin.

Ingredients:

1/2 teaspoon cider vinegar

2 tablespoons kaolin clay

1 teaspoon kukui nut or sweet almond oil

1 tablespoon sour cream or 1 egg yolk

1/2 teaspoon honey

1 drop neroli or palmarosa essential oil

2 drops sandalwood or rose essential oil

Directions:

1. Whisk together all ingredients in a small bowl, except the kaolin clay.

2. Stir in the clay, gradually until a paste of desired consistency is attained. Do not make it too thick.

3. Cleanse your face and neck area.

4. Apply the mask to your face and neck, while still damp, taking care to avoid eyes and mouth. Throw away any remainder.

5. Let it stay for 15 to 20 minutes.

6. Wash off with a wet and warm washcloth then apply a toner and moisturizer.

Turmeric Face Mask

For glowing Skin

Ingredients:

1/2 teaspoon turmeric powder

1/2 teaspoon organic apple cider vinegar

1/2 teaspoon milk or yogurt

1 tablespoon of organic, raw honey

1 drop lemon essential oil

Lemon oil (optional)

Directions:

1. Wash face and hands to remove any make-up.

2. Combine honey, turmeric powder, apple cider vinegar, yoghurt or milk or lemon oil, if using In a small jar, mixing well to attain a consistency that'll stick to your face.

3. Apply the mask gently avoiding your eyes. Leave it on for 15–20 minutes then rinse with warm water.

4. Cover and refrigerate any leftover.

5. Apply mask two times a week.

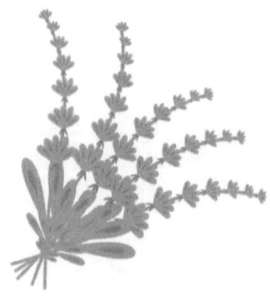

Face Mask For Acne And Oily Skin

A simple recipe to balance and deep- cleanse acne-prone and oily skin.

Ingredients:

3 teaspoons strong herbal tea or low fat yogurt

2 teaspoons cosmetic clay

1 drop tea tree essential oil

2 drops petitgrain or lemongrass essential oil

Directions:

1. Whisk together all ingredients in a small bowl.

2 Stir in enough tea or yogurt to create a paste of desired consistency. Do not make it too thick.

3. Cleanse your face and neck area.

4. While your skin is still damp, apply the mask to your face and neck, taking care to avoid eyes and mouth. Discard any remainder.

5. Leave it on your skin for 15-20 minutes.

6. Wash off with a warm and wet washcloth then apply a toner and moisturizer.

Acne Scar Face Mask

Remove those scars caused by acne with this recipe

Ingredients:

8–10 drops tea tree essential oil

6–8 drops helichrysum essential oil

8–10 drops frankincense essential oil

3 tablespoons lemon juice

3 tablespoons honey

2 tablespoons almond oil or olive oil

Directions:

1. Add together all ingredients in a jar and mix well.

2. Apply on skin and leave for 10–15 minutes then wash well.

3. Apply daily for about 8–10 days. Discontinue use if any discomfort occurs.

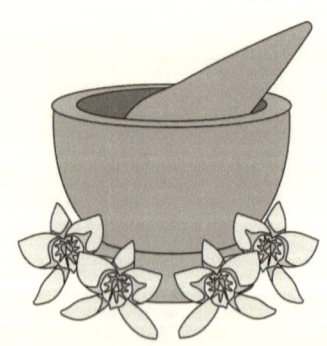

Face Mask For Sensitive And Problem Skin

Soothe and heal sensitive and problematic skin with this homemade face mask.

Ingredients:

Sensitive Skin Blend:

1/2 teaspoon Aloe Vera juice

1/2 tablespoon rolled oats

1/2 teaspoon evening primrose or avocado oil

1/2 tablespoon kaolin clay

1/2 teaspoon honey

 1/2 teaspoon milk or yogurt

1 drop rose or jasmine essential oil

1 drop lavender essential oil

1 drop chamomile essential oil

Psoriasis & Eczema Blend:

1/2 teaspoon Aloe Vera juice

1/2 teaspoon evening primrose or avocado oil

1/2 teaspoon honey

1/2 teaspoon milk or yogurt

1/2 tablespoon kaolin clay

1 drop helichrysum or chamomile essential oil

1 drop sandalwood or patchouli essential oil

1 drop rose or jasmine essential oil

Directions:

1. Grind the oats with a clean coffee grinder to attain a very smooth texture.

2. Whisk the Aloe Vera, oil and honey together.

3. Stir in the clay and oat powder, gradually until a paste of desired consistency is attained. Do not make it too thick.

3. Cleanse your face and neck area.

4. Apply the mask to your face and neck, while still damp, taking care to avoid eyes and mouth. Throw away any remainder.

5. Let it stay for 15 to 20 minutes.

6. Wash off with a wet and warm washcloth then apply a toner and moisturizer.

MASSAGE OIL RECIPES

Massage oils are relaxing and can be made any time you. They provide lubrication and enable your skin retain moisture. The oils are effortlessly absorbed by skin tissues to supply the desired therapeutic skin conditioning.

Sweet And Spicy Aphrodisiac Massage Oil

As the name suggest, this sensual massage oil works when you desire a nice night in with your partner.

Ingredients:

8 drops of sandalwood essential oil

2 drops patchouli essential oil

3 drops orange essential oil

1 drop ginger essential oil

1 drop ylang ylang essential oil

1/4 cup jojoba oil or apricot kernel oil

Directions:

1. Combine all the ingredients in a dark glass bottle.

2. Let it cure in a cool dark place for at least 24 hours.

3. Usage: Have a hot oil massage by heating the bottle in a bowl of hot water or you can simply have a full body massage.

4. Last up to 3 months.

Caution: if your skin is exceptionally sensitive, do not use ginger. Do not use prior to sun exposure because the lemon essential oil may cause sunburn.

Blissful Citrus Massage Oil

Enjoy the perfect remedy for depression.

Ingredients:

15 drops of bergamot essential oil

1/4 cup of jojoba oil apricot kernel oil

2 drops of ylang ylang essential oil

15 drops of palmarosa essential oil

Directions:

1. Combine all the ingredients in a dark glass bottle.

2. Let it cure in a cool dark place for at least 24 hours

3. Use it for a full body massage.

4. Shelf life is 3 months.

Caution: Do not use prior to sun exposure because the bergamot essential oil may cause sunburn.

Lavender Massage Oil

A pretty and beautifully scented oil that will provide healing for the body in many ways.

Ingredients:

12 drops of lavender essential oil

12 drops of orange essential oil

3 drops marjoram essential oil

2 drops clary sage essential oil

1 drop of vetiver essential oil

1/4 cup jojoba oil or sweet almond oil

Directions:

1. Combine all the ingredients in a dark glass bottle.

2. Let it cure in a cool dark place for at least 24 hours.

3. Use for a full body massage or rub on your chest, stomach and feet before bed for a good night rest.

4. Shelf life is 3 months.

Caution: Do not use prior to sun exposure because the orange essential oil may cause sunburn.

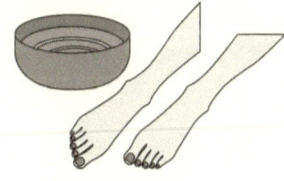

Lavender Massage Oil

Soothe your nerves and relax tight muscles with this recipe.

Ingredients:

8 drops of lavender essential oil

4 drops of marjoram essential oil

1 drop ginger essential oil

1 drop chamomile essential oil

1 drop cedarwood essential oil

1/4 cup jojoba oil or apricot kernel oil

Directions:

1. Combine all the ingredients in a dark glass bottle.

2. Let it cure in a cool dark place for at least 24 hours.

3. Use it for a full body massage.

4. Last up to 3 months.

Caution: Do not use ginger if your skin is exceptionally sensitive. Also leave out the chamomile if you are allergic to ragweed.

Stress Relief Aromatherapy Massage Oil

Bring relief to your body after a chaotic day with this recipe.

Ingredients:

5 drops frankincense essential oil

5 drops petitgrain essential oil

3 drops marjoram essential oil

1 drop vetiver essential oil

1 drop jasmine essential oil

1/4 cup jojoba oil or apricot kernel oil

Directions:

1. Combine all the ingredients in a dark glass bottle.

2. Let it cure in a cool dark place for at least 24 hours

3. Use for a full body massage or rub on your stomach, chest and feet just before bed for a good night rest. Also, rub on your temple during break time at work.

4. Shelf life is 3 months.

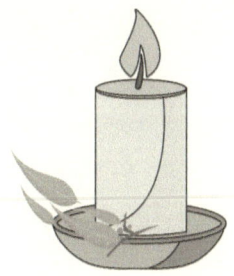

Anti-Snoring Massage Oil

This recipe contains ingredients with sedative properties that support breathing and helps the respiratory system to relax. Use it for a more relaxed sleep, even if you don't snore.

Ingredients:

4 drops marjoram essential oil

3 drops lemon essential oil

8 drops lavender essential oil

1/4 cup of sunflower oil or apricot kernel oil

Directions:

11. Combine all the ingredients in a dark glass bottle.

2. Let it cure in a cool dark place for at least 24 hours

3. Usage: Rub gently on the neck, upper chest and behind the ears.

4. Shelf life is 3 months.

Caution: Do not use prior to sun exposure because the lemon essential oil may cause sunburn.

FACIAL SKIN TONERS RECIPES

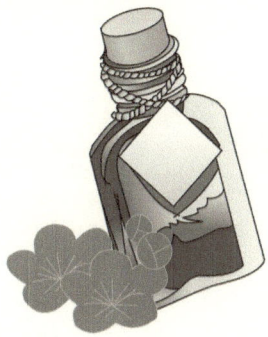

It is important to incorporate the use of a face toner in your skincare routine in order to boost the overall appearance of your skin. Besides, it helps to balance the oil production. A facial toner is also a quick way of giving your face its nightly beauty treatment when you are unable to cleanse your face properly before bed. You only need to spritz it on, wipe it off then apply a moisturizer.

Facial Skin Toner For Normal And Combination Skin
Ingredients:

1 drop patchouli essential oil

1 cup of rose geranium hydrosol

1 drop palmarosa essential oil

1 drop ylang ylang essential oil

1 drop rose geranium essential oil

7 drops lavender essential oil

Directions:

1. Combine all ingredients in a dark glass bottle and then shake well.

2. Leave it to cure for 24 hours, at least.

3. To use, shake the bottle, dip a cotton pad in the toner and wipe it over your face and neck area gently. Avoid your eyes.

4. Follow with a moisturizer or facial oil.

Facial Skin Toner For Mature, Dry And Sensitive Skin

This gentle anti-aging facial toner reduces wrinkles, soothes skin irritation and promotes healthy skin.

Ingredients:

1 cup of rose hydrosol

1 teaspoon of vegetable glycerin (optional)

3 drops frankincense essential oil

3 drops lavender essential oil

3 drops sandalwood essential oil

1 drop chamomile essential oil

Directions:

1. Combine all ingredients in a dark glass bottle and then shake well.

2. Leave it to cure for 24 hours, at least.

3. To use, shake the bottle, dip a cotton pad in the toner and wipe it over your face and neck area gently. Avoid your eyes.

4. Follow with a moisturizer or facial oil.

Facial Skin Toner For Acne And Oily Skin

This toner tightens pores, removes excess oil, and kills bacteria that cause acne.

Ingredients:

1 cup witch hazel

3 drops tea tree essential oil

3 drops palmarosa essential oil

3 drops lemongrass essential oil

1 drop rose geranium essential oil

3 drops petitgrain essential oil

Directions:

1. Combine all ingredients in a dark glass bottle and then shake well.

2. Leave it to cure for 24 hours, at least.

3. To use, shake the bottle, dip a cotton pad in the toner and wipe it over your face and neck area gently. Avoid your eyes.

4. Follow with a moisturizer or facial oil.

FACIAL SCRUBS RECIPES

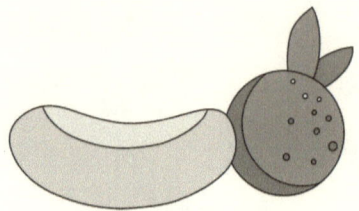

Recipes

Facial Scrub For Normal And Combination Skin
This facial scrub nourishes while scrubbing away dirt, dead skin cells and bacteria.

Ingredients:

2 cups rolled oats

1/2 cup almonds

2 tablespoons of dried lavender flowers

1/2 cup cosmetic clay

1/2 cup powdered milk

4 drops of lavender essential oil

2 drops frankincense essential oil

2 drops orange essential oil

1 drop rose geranium essential oil

1 drop roman chamomile essential oil

Directions:

90

1. Grind the oats, almonds and lavender flowers with a clean coffee grinder. Work in separate batches and ensure the oats and lavender flowers is grind very fine while the almond shouldn't be ground to powder. While grinding almonds, stop every now and then to test the texture by rubbing them between your fingers.

2. Combine the ground oats, lavender and almonds with clay and milk powder in a glass jar.

3. Add the essential oils, stirring properly to combine. Store the scrub in a cool, dark place.

4. <u>Usage:</u> mix 1heaping tablespoon with warm water, lotion or oil to create a paste.

5. Using gentle circular motions, massage the facial scrub into your face, taking care to avoid the eyes and mouth.

6. Let it on for 10 -15 minutes. Rinse off with warm water, pat dry and apply a toner and moisturizer.

Facial Scrub For Dry, Mature And Damaged Skin

Treat your face to the rejuvenating ability of this nourishing and healing scrub. It heals imperfections and reduces wrinkles.

Ingredients:

1/2 cup almonds

2 cups rolled oats

2 tablespoons dried rose petals (optional)

1/2 cup powdered milk

2 drops patchouli essential oil

4 drops frankincense essential oil

1 drop ylang ylang essential oil

1 drop helichrysum essential oil

2 drops sandalwood essential oil

Directions:

1. Grind the oats, almonds and lavender flowers with a clean coffee grinder. Work in separate batches and ensure the oats and lavender flowers is grind very fine while the almond shouldn't be ground to powder. While grinding almonds, stop every now and then to test the texture by rubbing them between your fingers.

2. Combine the ground oats, lavender and almonds with clay and milk powder in a glass jar.

3. Add the essential oils, stirring properly to combine. Store the scrub in a cool, dark place.

4. Usage: mix 1heaping tablespoon with warm water, lotion or oil to create a paste.

5. Using gentle circular motions, massage the facial scrub into your face, taking care to avoid the eyes and mouth.

6. Let it on for 10 -15 minutes. Rinse off with warm water, pat dry and apply a toner and moisturizer.

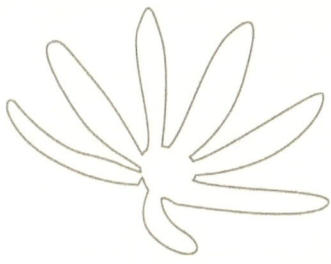

Scrub For Acne And Oily Skin

This is the best scrub for acne. It nourishes your skin, absorb excess oil, calms redness and cleanse away the dirt and grime.

Ingredients:

2 cups of quick cooking rolled oats

1/2 cup cornmeal

1/2 cup cosmetic clay

3 drops lavender essential oil

1 drop rose geranium essential oil

4 drops lemongrass essential oil

2 drops tea tree essential oil

Directions:

1. Grind the oats, almonds and lavender flowers with a clean coffee grinder. Work in separate batches and ensure the oats and lavender flowers is grind very fine while the almond shouldn't be ground to powder. While grinding almonds, stop every now and then to test the texture by rubbing them between your fingers.

2. Combine the ground oats, lavender and almonds with clay and milk powder in a glass jar.

3. Add the essential oils, stirring properly to combine. Store the scrub in a cool, dark place.

4. <u>Usage:</u> mix 1 heaping tablespoon with warm water, lotion or oil to create a paste.

5. Using gentle circular motions, massage the facial scrub into your face, taking care to avoid the eyes and mouth.

6. Let it on for 10 -15 minutes. Rinse off with warm water, pat dry and apply a toner and moisturizer.

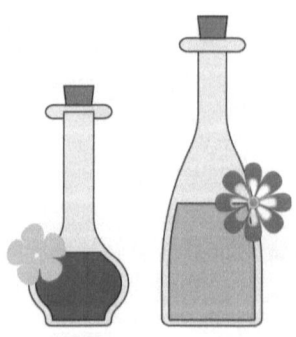

SOAP RECIPES
(Soaps, lotion bars & Body Washes)

Homemade soap recipes are safer and more cost-effective. Essential oils added to the ingredients provide therapeutic and purifying benefits.

Recipes

Silky Body Wash
Ingredients:

1 tbsp Shea butter

1/4 cup Aloe Vera gel

3/4 tsp Guar gum

3/4 cup Castile Soap

25 drops Essential oils of choice

Directions:

1. Add the Shea butter to a pan and melt on low heat. Add the aloe Vera gel to the Shea butter and warm together.

2. Now add the gum and use a whisk to stir thoroughly and then add in the soap base.

3. Mix thoroughly in a blender to get the gum fully distributed. Your wash will appear foamy but will settle in a couple of hours.

4. Pour some in your bath or use in the shower.

Homemade Lemon Soap

Ingredients:

13 cubes Goat's milk soap base

Lemon essential oil

3-4 lemons of Lemon zest (optional)

Directions:

1. Cut the soap into cubes.

2. Melt soap for about 2 minutes using a large pyrex measuring cup.

3. As soon as soap cubes turn liquid, add the lemon zest and some drops of the lemon essential oil and stir well.

4. Pour into soap molds. Leave for one hour to harden.

5. Press mold to release soap.

Hand Wash Liquid Soap

Ingredients:

1 cup Liquid Soap

1 cup Water

8 drops Essential oils of choice

Directions:

1. Mix ingredients together.

2. Pour into a bottle and shake thoroughly.

Seaweed Soap

Ingredients:

32 ounces Clear soap base

6-8 pieces dried seaweed

1 teaspoon extra virgin olive oil

1.5 teaspoons Lemon essential oil

1 teaspoon Lavender essential oil

Dash of green mica

Mold: 3 part Ziploc, divided rectangle mold

Directions:

1. Place seaweed pieces into mold.

2. Slice the soap base into tiny cubes.

3. Add the essential oils, colorant and olive oil just before the soap is completely melted, stir well.

4. Slowly pour into the molds. Leave soap in freezer or fridge to harden. It may remain in at room temperature, however.

5. Remove from molds. Once the soap is at room temperature, cut and wrap.

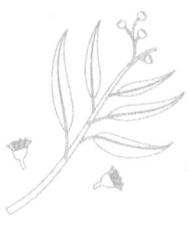

Antibacterial & Antiviral Hand Wash Soap

Ingredients:

1 cup Liquid Soap

1 cup Water

8 drops essential oils of choice

3 drops Tea Tree oil

5 drops Lavender oil

Directions:

1. Mix ingredients together.

2. Pour into a bottle and shake thoroughly

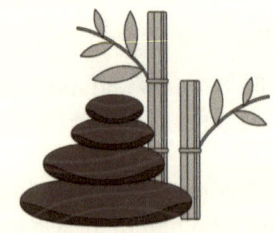

Sweet Honey Soap

Ingredients:

1 lb Castile soap

1/4 lb Honey

1/4 lb Glycerin

5drops Sandalwood essential oil

2 tbsp Fine oatmeal

Directions:

1. Grate the soap.

2. Put some water in the pot and add the honey, glycerin, the oatmeal and essential oil, mixing well until soap is dissolved.

3. Boil for 3 minutes, pour into soap moulds or a deep wet container. Cut into pieces when it is quite cold.

4. Leave out until it's dry before storing.

Lavender Soap

Ingredients:

1 soap, unscented

1dried lavender

3 drops Lavender essential oil

Directions:

1. Grate a bar unscented soap and place inside some water in a bowl.

2. Place the bowl in a pan of hot water. Stir thoroughly until smooth then add the dried lavender flowers to the soap.

3. Remove the bowl from pan. Add lavender essential oil and pour into molds.

Simple Soap Recipe

Ingredients:

1 lb Castile Soap Flakes and or/Glycerin Soap

8 drops Fennel essential oil

14 drops Grapefruit essential oil

8 drops Lemon essential oil

1 cup Purified Water

1/2 cup Herbal Tea or Hydrosol

Directions:

1. Melt the glycerin in double boiler hydrosol or herbal infusion then set aside to cool for a while.

2. Add essential oil and stir thoroughly. Pour into moulds and leave to harden.

3. Once hardened, cut into bars, using a knife to smooth rough spots.

Herbal Soap

Ingredients:

1g Block olive or veg. soap

25 g herbs, loosely chopped

3 drops Thyme or rosemary essential oil

1 tbsp finely ground oatmeal

Directions:

1. Grate the soap into a bowl and add the remaining ingredients. Heat gently till it melts and then mix well.

2. Pour soup into each section of an egg box that has been lined with waxed paper.

Basic Lotion Bars

Ingredients:

2 oz Beeswax

1 oz Almond oil

1 oz Cocoa butter

3drops Essential oil

Directions:

1. Melt cocoa butter and beeswax and on the stove in a clean pot.

2. Once it melts, remove from heat and then add the almond oil.

3. Mix in the essential oil drop by drop until it's attains the desired scent.

4. Pour the mixture into a mould. Leave it to it set fully before using.

Lemon/ Cedar Men's Body Wash

Bubbly with the perfect consistency, these men's body wash will leave you moisturized after a shower. You wouldn't even need to apply a moisturizer or lotion or afterwards!

Ingredients

1/2 cup distilled water

1 cup Castile liquid soap

1 Cup of fractionated coconut oil/ almond oil mix

1 tsp salt (for preservation)

1 tsp of kosher/epsom salt (for a longer shelf life)

20 drops of lemongrass oil essential oil

10 drops of cedar wood oil essential oil

Super Aromatic Men's Body Wash
Ingredients

1/2 cup distilled water

1 cup Castile liquid soap

1 cup of fractionated coconut oil/ almond oil mix

1 tsp salt (for preservation)

1 tsp of kosher/Epsom salt (for a longer shelf life)

15 drops lavender essential oil

10 drops patchouli essential oil

5 drops clary sage essential oil

Sweet & Strong Men's Body Wash

Ingredients

1/2 cup distilled water

1 cup Castile liquid soap

1 cup of fractionated coconut oil/ almond oil mix

1 tsp salt (for preservation)

1 tsp of kosher/Epsom salt (for a longer shelf life)

10 drops sweet orange essential oil

10 drops patchouli essential oil

10 drops lavender essential oil

Directions For All Three:

1. Combine all ingredients into a bottle, and shake thoroughly.

2. Store leftovers in mason jars for refills.

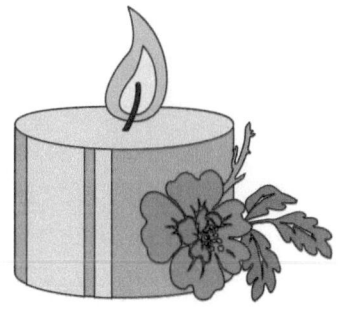

HAIR CARE RECIPES

Several hair growth care and treatments depend on essential oils. Essential oils are versatile and can work wonders on any type of hair and scalp. Some of them work directly on the hair by helping to strengthen and repair it. Others help to improve the condition of the scalp alone.

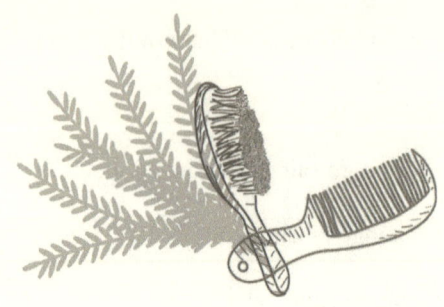

Avocado Hair Moisturizing

Ingredients:

Half avocado

Few drops Peppermint essential oil

1-2 tbsp Oil (optional)

1-2 tbsp Egg yolk (optional)

Directions:

1. Mash the avocado up and then add the essential oil.

2. Shampoo your hair, squeeze the water out and apply mask. Allow to sit for 15minutes then rinse off afterwards.

3. Hair will come out super soft and smell real nice.

Homemade Hair Softener/ Growth

This recipe promotes hair growth and softens hair.

Ingredients:

2 drops Thyme essential oil

2 drops Cedar essential oil

3 drops Rosemary essential oil

1 ounce Grapeseed

1 tbsp Jojoba

Directions:

1. Mix all the ingredients in a bowl. Pour into a tight bottle for easy storage.

2. Every night, massage the mixture into your scalp and rinse in cool water and shampoo the next morning.

3. For oily hair, 3 times in a week is fine.

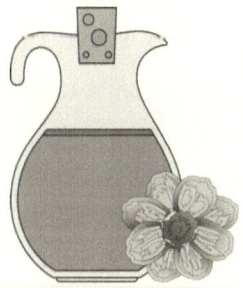

Lavender/ Rosemary Hair Spray

Hair spray helps to set the hair and prevent fly away. Eliminate toxins and enjoy a beautiful and healthy hair by making yours using this recipe.

Ingredients:

1 cup boiled and filtered water

1 tablespoon vodka

2 tablespoons cane sugar

10 drops rosemary essential oil

10 drops lavender essential oil

Directions:

1. Add sugar to boiled water to dissolve then stir.

2. Add the vodka, blend once more and let it cool for a while.

3. Add the essential oils and blend well.

4. Place mixture in a glass spray bottle and store in a cool place. Shake before use. This mixture serves 30.

Note: Lavender and Rosemary essential oils help with hair loss. While spraying, do not let it get into your eyes or mouth.

Split Ends Remedy
Ingredients:

10 drops Sandalwood essential oil

10 drops Rosemary essential oil

Directions:

1. Combine ingredients

2. Use your fingers to rub them in.

Warm Oil Recipe For Dry Hair
Ingredients:

2 ounces Aloe Vera gel

2 ounces Castor oil

6 drops Rose geranium cedar essential oil

8 drops Rosemary essential oil

2 drops Ginger essential oil

Directions:

1. Combine all the ingredients.

2. Warm the mixture and apply to scalp and hair in sections

3. Use a towel to cover the head and leave it on for an hour. Wash off.

Itchy Scalp Shampoo Recipe

Ingredients:

10 drops of rosemary essential oil

2 tablespoons apple cider vinegar

1 tablespoon raw honey

4 ounces aloe vera gel

1 teaspoon Castile soap

1 tablespoon coconut oil

3 tablespoons of purified or filtered water

10 drops of tea tree essential oil

Directions:

1. Add together the honey and apple cider vinegar. Add the aloe vera and coconut oil, blending well.

2. Once dissolved, place in a mixing bowl.

3. Add the castile soap and water then blend. Add the essential oils and blend once again.

4. Pour into bottle, tightly cap and shake well. Wet hair and apply, gently massaging into the scalp, rinsing well.

5. This makes 6 ounces

Note: Tea tree oil is so versatile because it has natural antifungal, anti-inflammatory and antibacterial properties, which are all good for an itchy scalp. It is so gentle it can be used every day too. Rosemary essential oil helps to thicken your hair and even prevent baldness.

After Shampooing Rinse: For Dry Hair
Ingredients:

2 tsp Comfrey oil

2 tsp Marshmallow oil

2 drops Parsley essential oil

2 drops Sage essential oil

4 cups Water

2cups Vinegar

Directions:

1. Combine all the ingredients. Rinse your hair with this mixture after shampooing.

2. Keep it away from your eyes.

3. Reuse rinse once or twice.

Sweet-Smelling Herbal Shampoo
Ingredients:

2 ounces Unscented shampoo

12 drops Chamomile essential oil

12 drops Lavender essential oil

Directions:

1. Mix all the ingredients

2. Shake well before use.

Henna Protein Treatment

Ingredients:

3 ounces Henna

2 tbsp Honey

24 drops Lavender essential oil

2 cups Warm water

1 tsp Olive oil

1Egg

Directions:

1. Mix all the ingredients. Add this mixture to henna, remove any lumps.

2. Wet the hair and apply from roots to ends.

3. Keep the heat in by covering for 1 or 2 hours with a plastic bag and towel

4. The henna breaks down and the color becomes darker when you do this but ensure that the henna doesn't dry out.

5. Rinse several times with warm water, and then apply shampoo and conditioner to it.

6. Make sure you use gloves and wear an apron to avoid staining your skin.

Deep Endings Essential Oil Treatment

The ends of your hair will be nourished by this revitalizing oil treatment. Its usefulness is more pronounced in the winter when hair tends to rub up against heavy fabrics, including wools.

Ingredients:

1-3 tsp Sweet almond, olive or peanut oil

2-4 drops lavender essential oil

<u>Note:</u>

The quantity of the peanut, olive or sweet almond oil depends on how long or thick your hair is.

Directions:

1. Combine the oils and apply it to the end of your hair.

2. Using a clear plastic wrap, wrap the hair and leave for about 30 minutes.

3. Rinse with Lemon Aid.

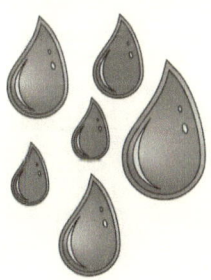

Dry Scalp Remedy With Rosemary Oil

Ingredients:

6 drops tea tree oil

8 drops cedarwood oil

8 drops rosemary oil

1 teaspoon raw honey

4 ounces olive oil, coconut or almond oil

Directions:

1. Add all ingredients together in a glass container, mixing well.

2. Massage into the scalp and leave on for 20-30 minutes. (For severe conditions, leave overnight.)

3. Shampoo thoroughly. Use 2 or 3 times

Lavender Mist

Lavender helps to cleanse and revive your hair.

Ingredients:

½ gallon water

5 drops lavender essential oil

Directions:

1. Pour the half gallon of water in a large pot.

2. Cover, boil and let it simmer for 1 hour so as to remove impurities.(Distilled water can also be used).

3. Remove from heat and then add the lavender oil. Stir thoroughly, leave to cool

4. Pour into spritz bottles

Homemade Hair Conditioner Oil

Ingredients:

3 drops Rosemary essential oil

1 tablespoon Jojoba oil

Directions:

1. Mix the essential oil (Rosemary) and jojoba in a small bow

2. Wet your hair with warm water, apply the mixture and leave it to sit on your hair for 30 minutes.

3. Wash your hair afterwards.

Scaly Scalp And Dandruff Blend

<u>Ingredients:</u>

2 drops Atlas cedar- wood

2 drops Rosemary

2 drops Lavender

2 drops Tea tree oil

1/2 ounce Jojoba

<u>Directions:</u>

1. Mix all ingredients together.

2. Apply on scalp

Scented Hair Gel

<u>Ingredients:</u>

1 cup Water

2 tbsp Flax seed

2 drops Essential oil

<u>Directions:</u>

1. In a small saucepan, mix water and seed. Bring to boil and then remove from heat.

2. Allow to set for 30 minutes and then strain. Once cooled, add essential oil

3. Pour into to a wide-mouthed container with lid.

Quality Hair Treatment

This recipe is ideal for a thicker, smoother and nice- smelling hair.

Ingredients:

2 spoons Honey

2 spoons Olive oil

2 Eggs

10 drops Rose EO

5 drops Lavender EO

Directions:

1. Combine all ingredients

2. Apply all over the hair.

3. Leave for an hour then wash away.

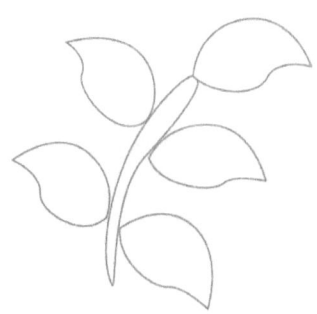

LIPS AND MOUTH CARE RECIPES
(Lip balms, Lip gloss, Lip scrubs & Tooth whitener)

True; dry, cracked lips do not do our face much harm. But there's no need applying toxic chemicals onto our skin and mouth when we can just make ours safely and cheaply. Nourish and hydrate your lips by making your own lip balms. Use Vitamin E as a preservative. Nevertheless, throw away all homemade Lip Balms once it changes color and odor.

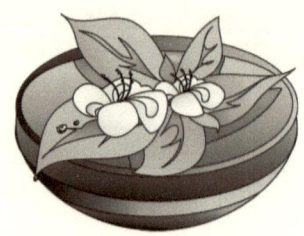

Pomegranate Lip Balm
Ingredients:

2 tablespoons of bees wax

1 tablespoon olive oil

1 teaspoon coconut oil

1 tsp honey

7 drops of pomegranate oil

Lip balm tins or tubes

Directions:

1. Melt beeswax, olive oil and coconut oil in a pot over medium low heat and stir with wooden spoon or chopstick. Remove from heat

2. Add honey and pomegranate oil, whisking thoroughly to distribute the oils.

3. Pour quickly into balm tins or jars. Let it cool to harden.

4. This recipe serves 3-6 lip balm tins.

Honey Cocoa Lip Balm

Ingredients:

2 tsp Olive oil

½ tsp Cocoa butter

½ tsp Honey

½ tsp Beeswax

3 drops Orange essential oil

1Vitamin E capsule

Directions:

1. Place the cocoa butter, oil and beeswax into a glass pan. melt over low heat with hotplate.

2. Stir until thoroughly melted. Remove from heat

3. Add the honey and essential oil into it. Squeeze the vitamin E capsule into the mixture and stir.

4. Pour the mixture into fine containers.

Honey Balm

Ingredients:

3 oz almond oil

½ oz. Beeswax or Beeswax Pellets

2 teaspoons honey

1-4 drops essential Oil

1Vitamin E capsule

Directions:

1. Mix the beeswax and almond oil together in a bowl.

2. Place bowl in a pan of water and heat on a stovetop.

3. Heat until mixture is fully melted, stirring continuously to completely melt the wax.

4. Remove from heat and add the honey and essential oil in it.

5. Open the vitamin E capsule, squeeze the contents into it. Stir the mixture one more time

6. Allow it to completely cool. Once cool, pour mixture into small plastic containers.

Peppermint Lip Balm

Protect and pamper and your lips with recipe when the weather turns dry.

Ingredients:

2 tbsp Petroleum jelly

1 tsp Beeswax

10-14 drops Peppermint essential oil

Directions:

1. Melt the petroleum jelly in a small pot. Add in the beeswax and then remove from the heat once melted.

2. Now add the peppermint essential oil

3. Pour into a lip pot and leave to cool.

Natural Teeth Whitener

Get your smile back with this natural teeth whitener recipe. it cleanses and works real well!

Ingredients:

3 drops lemon essential oil

1 teaspoon of baking soda

1 mashed strawberry

Directions:

1. Combine baking soda and strawberry until it forms a paste.

2. Add the essential oil drops. Apply paste mixture on your toothbrush and brush teeth for a minute or two.

3. Rinse mouth and brush teeth again with your normal tooth paste.

4. Refrigerate leftover for 1 to 3 days. Shake well before each use.

Natural Toothpaste

Ingredients:

25 drops of peppermint essential oil

3 tablespoons coconut oil

1 packet stevia

3 tablespoons baking soda

2 teaspoon vegetable glycerin

Directions:

1. In a jar, mash together the baking soda and coconut oil

2. Add in the other ingredients to form a paste.

3. Cover tightly and store.

4. Dip in your toothbrush to use.

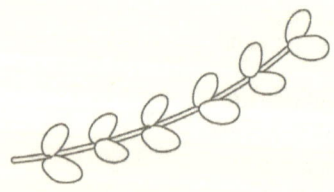

Lavender Lemon Lip Balm

Ingredients:

4 tbsp coconut oil

3 tbsp Bees wax

7 drops lemon essential oil

7 drops lavender essential oil

2 drops Vitamin E

Directions:

1. Melt beeswax, olive oil, vitamin E and coconut oil in a pot over medium low heat and stir with wooden spoon or chopstick. Remove from heat.

2. Add the essential oils, whisking thoroughly to distribute the oils all through the mixture.

3. Pour quickly into balm tins or jars. Let it cool to harden.

4. This recipe serves 2-3 lip balm tins.

Note: Use glass or tin containers to store citrus essentials oils such as Lemon, on account of their highly concentrated and acidic properties.

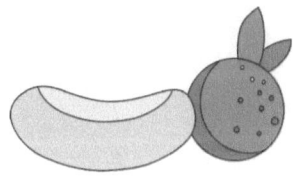

Tangerine Lip Gloss
Ingredients:

2 tsp Beeswax

1 tsp Honey

7 tsp Sweet almond, jojoba or castor oil

5 drops tangerine essential oil

Directions:

1. Melt the beeswax and oil until completely melted.

2. Remove from heat and then add the honey, whisking all together.

3. When the mixture is almost cool, add the essential oil and mix it up again.

4. Pour into a container.

Lemon Lip Gloss
Ingredients:

2 tsp beeswax

1 tsp honey

7 tsp sweet almond, jojoba or castor oil

5 drops Lemon essential oil

 Directions:

1. Melt the beeswax and oil until completely melted.

2. Remove from heat and then add the honey, whisking all together.

3. When the mixture is almost cool, add the essential oil and mix it up again.

4. Pour into a container. To make it harder, add more beeswax

Hemp Oil Lip Balm
Ingredients:

3 tbsp coconut oil

Castor oil

1 tbsp Sunflower oil

1 tbsp Hemp seed oil

1 tbsp Beeswax

1 tbsp Honey

Few drops Peppermint essential oil

Directions:

1. Melt the coconut oil and wax together. Add the honey and heat for some time.

2. Stir continuously and add the sunflower and castor oil.

3. As the mixture thickens, add the peppermint essential oil and the hempseed oil. Stir until it thickens.

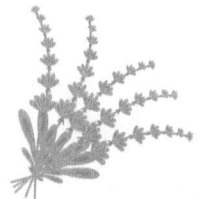

Rose-Coco Lip Balm
Ingredients:

2 Tbsp coconut oil

1 Tbsp grated cocoa butter

1 Tbsp dried rosebuds (or any dried flower)

1/4 tsp Vitamin E oil

3 drops Rose, vanilla or lavender essential oil

Directions:

1. Place the coconut oil in a stainless steel bowl and melt over very low heat.

2. Once melted, add the roses (or any dried flowers of your choice) and stir thoroughly. Place on very low heat again for an hour.

3. Use a cheesecloth or fine-mesh sieve to sieve the oil into a bowl. Clean your original heating bowl and pour the oil back in. Return to heat.

4. Add the cocoa butter and stir until well melted. Remove from heat.

5. Add essential oil and vitamin E oil and stir well. Transfer to a container and leave it for 3 hours to set.

Note:

Remember, this is mostly coconut oil, so do not put this recipe in a lip balm tube. Do not keep in your pocket, either. Coconut oil liquefies quickly when it is in contact with only a small amount of heat. Even keeping it in a warm place like your body will make it leak all over.

Minty Choc Lip Balm

Ingredients:

1 Tbsp Beeswax pearls or grated beeswax

1/8 cup Coconut oil

1/2 Tbsp Shear butter

1/2 Tbsp Cocoa butter

1/2 tsp Honey

1 tsp Cocoa powder

1/8 tsp Vitamin E oil

3 drops Peppermint essential oil

Directions:

1. In a small pot, place the cocoa and Shea butters and add the coconut oil.

2. Heat over extremely low heat for 20 minutes. Stir occasionally. (Do not let the mixture go beyond 175 degrees else the Shea butter will become a little gritty.)

3. Add in the beeswax and stir and remove from heat once completely melted.

4. Add the honey, cocoa powder, essential oil, and vitamin E, whisking thoroughly the whole time.

5. Once everything is incorporated, transfer to a lip balm tin and leave for 3hours to set.

Sweet Lavender Lip Balm
Ingredients:

1 tbsp Beeswax pearls or grated beeswax

1 tsp Honey

1 tsp Cocoa powder (optional)

J4 tbsp jojoba, olive or almond oil

1/4 tsp Vitamin E oil

7 drops Lavender essential oil

1 tsp Colored, natural lipstick to give it a hint of color (optional)

Directions:

1. Warm the honey, oils and beeswax on very low heat in a small bowl.

2. Stir until the beeswax is totally melted. Remove from heat.

3. Quickly whisk in the colored lipstick, cocoa powder, essential oil and vitamin E.

4. Place the bowl into a pan of ice water and keep on whisking as you add the honey.

5. Once the honey is fully incorporated, transfer the balm quickly into your lip balm container

6. Leave to set for 3 hours.

Note

Mineral eye shadow tubs make great lip balm containers so do not throw yours away after use. It's fun to be creative. Match and mix colors until you find the one you love.

Cold Sores Treatment Lip Balm
Ingredients:

1 oz emu oil

1 oz almond oil

1 oz avocado oil

1 /2 oz. beeswax pellets or shaved beeswax

1/4 oz Aloe Vera Gel

6 drops lavender essential oil

2 drops tea tree essential oil

3 drops lime essential oil

Directions:

1. Mix the beeswax, emu, almond and avocado oil together in a bowl.

2. Heat the bowl in a pan of water on a stove. Stir the mixture repeatedly until the beeswax is melted.

3. Add the aloe Vera gel. Remove from heat, add the essential oils and stir.

4. Stir once more and leave to completely cool. Transfer into small plastic tins when cool.

Sweet Sugar Lip Balm
Ingredients:

20 ml Sweet almond oil

½ tsp Grated beeswax or beeswax pellets

½ tsp Cocoa butter

1 tsp icing sugar

1 capsule Vitamin E

5 drops Peppermint, sweet orange or rose essential oil

Directions:

1. Melt cocoa butter, beeswax and oil in a double boiler. Add the icing sugar and stir so it dissolves.

2. Remove from heat and then add the vitamin E by puncturing the capsule and pouring oil in.

3. Add the essential oils, stir again and pour into a lip balm container.

Luscious Lip Balm

Ingredients:

1 tbsp (0.5 oz) Filtered, raw beeswax

4 tbsp Unscented coconut oil

10 drops Bergamot essential oil

Directions:

1. Add beeswax and coconut oil to a glass measuring cup.

2. Microwave every 30 second until beeswax is melted. Remove the mixture from the microwave and set aside

3. Add the essential oil to the mixture, stirring carefully. Pour slowly into your lip balm tins.

4. Leave at room temperature to cool and set.

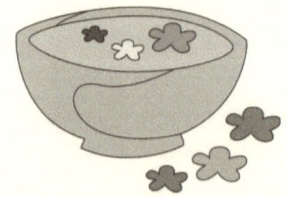

NAIL CARE RECIPES

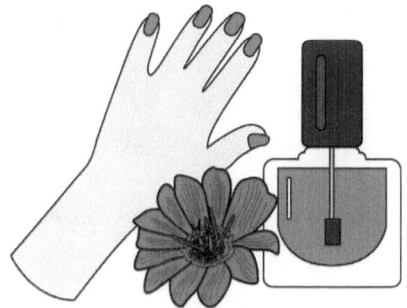

Nail Growth Soak

Ingredients:

4 drops rosemary essential oil

1/4 cup coconut oil

1/4 cup raw honey

Directions:

1. Combine all the ingredients in a bowl.

2. Put it in the microwave for 20 seconds.

3. Once warmed, soak your hands for about 15 minutes.

4. Repeat two times in a week.

Nail Moisturizing Soak

Ingredients:

4 drops lavender essential oil

1 tablespoon hemp seed Oil

Directions:

1. Combine all the ingredients in a bowl.

2. Soak your nails in it for 15-18 minutes. Rinse well

Anti-Aging Hand Oil

Ingredients:

3 drops carrot seed essential oil

6 tablespoons jojoba oil

3 drops pomegranate extract

2 tablespoons flax seed oil

Directions:

1. Add together all ingredients in a bowl.

2. Apply mixture to your hands then cover them with zip lock bags.

3. Let it stay for 20 minutes then take off and wash hands.

4. Use several times in a week.

DEODORANTS AND POWDERS

(Foundations, powders and deodorants)

A lot of people react very strongly to store-bought deodorant. Homemade deodorants are a healthy alternative and they cost much less as well.

Simple Deodorant Powder

Ingredients:

3tbsp Coconut Oil

3tbsp Baking Soda

2tbsp Shea Butter

2tbsp Arrowroot

5drop Essential Oils

Directions:

1. Melt coconut oil and Shea butter in a double boiler over low heat until barely melted. Remove from heat.

2. Add arrowroot and baking soda, mixing well.

3. Add essential oils and pour into a glass container for storage.

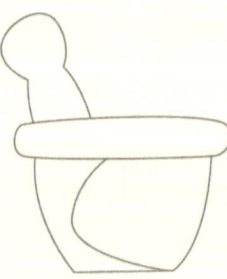

Pineapple Deodorant Powder

Ingredients

1 tbsp Coconut oil

1 cup Baking soda

1/2 cups powdered coconut milk

1 tbsp Pineapple essential oil

Directions

1. Melt coconut oil and set aside.

2. Mix coconut powder and baking soda in a tight-lid container.

3. Add essential oil and the melted coconut oil.

4. Use a powder brush or puff to apply the deodorant.

Scented Orange Deodorant Powder

Ingredients:

3 tsp Baking soda

2tbsp Arrowroot powder

2tbsp Cornflour

10 drops Sweet orange essential oil

10 drops Neroli essential oil

Directions:

1. Mix all the dry ingredients in bowl.

2. Add the essential oils, mix well. Store in an airtight container.

Fine Thyme Deodorant Powder

Ingredients:

1 1/2 cup Arrowroot

Baking soda/ bicarbonate of soda

1/4 cup Finely powdered thyme

1/4 cup Calcium bentonite clay

1 tbsp Zeolite powder

100 drops Rosemary essential oil

50 drops Thyme essential oil

Directions

1. Combine all the ingredients except the essential oils in a large bowl.

2. Blend in a food processor for 20 seconds or whisk by hand.

3. Slowly add the essential oils to 7 tablespoons of the powder mix. Use a mortar and pestle.

4. Add oil mixture to the rest of the powder and whirl for 20 seconds in a food processor.

5. Let the mixture sit for 3 days so that the oils can permeate the powder.

6. Place in a small jar.

Face Powder Foundation

Ingredients

2 tbsp Cornstarch or arrowroot powder

1½ tsp or more Cinnamon, nutmeg or cocoa powder

5 drops Essential oil

Directions

1. Mix all the ingredients in a bowl. Stir until well mixed.

2. Add tint (cocoa powder, cinnamon or nutmeg) until you attain your desired color.

3. Keep adding any of these tints until you get a similar tone for your skin.

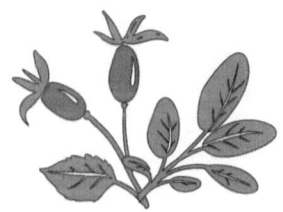

Homemade Probiotic Deodorant

Ingredients:

1 tbsp Cocoa butter

1 tbsp Coconut oil

1 tbsp Shea butter

1 tbsp Beeswax

2 1/2 tbsp Arrowroot powder

1 tbsp Baking soda

1/4 tsp Vitamin E oil

15 drops Essential oils of choice

2 capsules powdered probiotics

Directions

1. Melt the Shea butter, beesawax, coconut oil and cocoa butter over very low heat.

2. Remove from heat then add the baking soda and arrowroot powder to it.

3. Whisk until all powders are dissolved and mixed.

4. Add essential oils and vitamin E oil. Cool mixture.

5. Once it is cooled, open the capsules of probiotics and add powder to the mixture, stirring quickly with spatula to combine

6. Add mixture to used but clean deodorant container.

7. Place in refrigerator to cool and harden.

8. Store afterwards. Shelf-life is for 3-4 months.

Herbal Deodorant Powder
Ingredients:

2 parts powdered sandalwood

1 part powdered white oak bark

1 part powdered lovage root

Directions:

1. Pulverize herbs in a food processor or blender until they are in powdered form.

2. Transfer powder into an iron skillet. Pan-roast gently.

3. Pour powdered herbs into a muslin draw-string bags.

4. Pat bags on your feet or under your arms.

Sage Deodorizing Powder
For Foot

Ingredients:

1 tbsp Baking powder

2 drops Sage essential oil

Directions:

1. Mix oil and baking powder in a plastic bag. Shake thoroughly. Set aside to dry.

2. Break up any formed clumps.

3. Use powder to regularly dust feet

4. Leave a teaspoon in the shoes overnight.

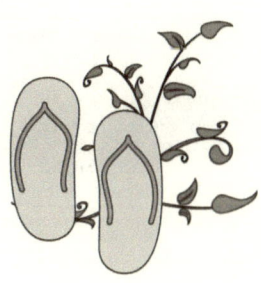

Fairy Dusting Powder

Ingredients:

1/2 cup Rice Flour

1/2 cup Cornstarch

2 tsp Finely ground Rose petals

1/2 tsp Mica, very fine glitter

3 drops Essential Oil

Directions:

1. Mix all the dry ingredients together

2. Add essential oil and mix thoroughly

3. Put in an airtight container

Lemony Deodorant

Ingredients:

1-1/3 cups of Extra virgin coconut oil

1-1/2 tablespoons of Beeswax shavings

3/4 cup Arrowroot powder

2 tbsp Clay

25 drops Tea tree essential oil

5 drops Lemongrass essential oil

1/4 cup of Baking soda

Directions:

1. Melt beeswax and coconut oil over low heat until barely melted.

2. Remove from heat and then add the remaining ingredients apart from essential oils.

3. Leave to cool while stirring continuously until it hardens.

4. Refrigerate to speed this up. Check and stir frequently.

5. Add essential oils and thoroughly combine.

6. Pour into empty deodorant containers.

7. Leave in a cool location or refrigerate to harden.

8. For each arm, use about 1/8 teaspoon.

Simply Fresh Deodorant Powder

Ingredients:

6 tbsp Coconut oil

4 tbsp Baking soda

4 tbsp Arrowroot or cornstarch

5 drops Essential oils

Directions:

1. In a medium sized bowl, mix arrowroot and baking soda together.

2. Use a fork to mash in coconut oil until well mixed. Add essential oil

3. Store in a used deodorant container for easy use.

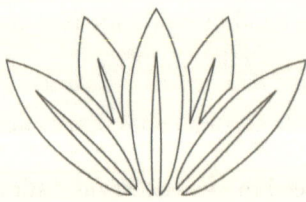

LOTION, SHEA BUTTER AND OIL RECIPES

(Body lotions, Shear butters, face lotions, sprays & oils)

Egyptian history records how its royalties cared for their hair, skin and body with all- natural homemade products. Their queens were beautiful, with radiant skin and a glowing complexion. And this was made possible with natural lotions; not chemical-laden ones.

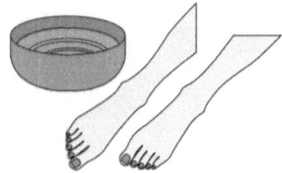

The benefits of making and using natural products of which include natural body lotions are numerous. Let's highlight a few:

1. You will know the ingredients that soothe your skin.

2. There is zero risk of skin irritation.

3. They don't clog pores and they let the skin breathe naturally.

4. They do not cause acne or eczema.

5. They are environmental friendly – all the natural ingredients used (oils, butters, herbs) are biodegradable and won't harm the nature, as nature itself provides them.

6. They do not affect your pets through accidental sniffing or licking. They are totally safe in the home.

7. They are inexpensive. They cost a lot less than cosmetic products. This is because once you have discovered what kind of butters and oils suit your skin, you can purchase them in bulk and by doing this, you get to save a great amount of money.

8. It enhances creativity. Your preferred combination can be prepared with a little creativity on your part.

9. You get to use only the fragrances you enjoy due to the wide range of essential oils.

Recipes

Non-Greasy Moisturizing Lotion

Ingredients:

1 cup Aloe Vera gel

1 tsp Vitamin E oil

1½ tbsp Grated beeswax

1/2 cup Almond or grape-seed oil

1tbsp Cocoa butter (optional)

10 drops Essential oils of choice

Note:

Beeswax is used for thickening creams.

Directions:

1. Melt beeswax and oils in a double boiler over low heat.

2. Combine aloe Vera gel and vitamin E oil in a medium-sized bowl.

3. Pour the melted oils into a blender. Leave to cool at room temperature.

4. Once cooled, add the essential oils, put the blender on low speed and slowly pour in the aloe Vera mixture.

5. Blend the mixture until it looks and feel like lotion. Pour the lotion into clean jars.

6. It will last 6 weeks when refrigerated, less without.

Uplifting Homemade Lotion

Suitable for very dry skin, this lotion moisturizes and nourishes when used regularly.

Ingredients

1/8 cup coconut oil

1/4 cup cocoa butter

1/8 cup sweet almond oil

50 drops Orange essential oil

Note:

Cocoa Butter is one of the most stable fats containing natural antioxidants and moisturizers, making it ideal for the prevention and removal of stretch marks.

It absorbs quickly into the skin and is used as an active ingredient in most creams for stretch marks, eczema or dermatitis. Cocoa butter creates a barrier for sensitive skin, protecting it from external factors and maintaining moisture levels.

Directions

1. Use a double boiler to melt the oils and the cocoa butter.

2. Remove from heat and place in the freezer for 15-20 minutes until it begins to harden.

3. Add the essential oil and use a hand mixer to beat the mixture until smooth.

4. Store in a dry, clean jar.

Easy Lotion

Ingredients:

1 cup olive oil

8 tbsp coconut oil

8 tbsp beeswax, pastilles

1/2 tsp vitamin E oil

20 drops essential oil

Directions:

1. Combine beeswax pastilles, olive oil and coconut oil in a jar.

2. Put the jar into a saucepan and then fill the saucepan with water, ¾ all the way up the jar. (Be careful, the water mustn't get into the oil mixture).

3. Heat and stir on the stove over low heat until it melts. Leave to cool at room temperature or refrigerated.

4. Add in the essential oil and Vitamin E.

5. While it's cooling, use a fork to stir thoroughly every 15 minutes.

Coconut &Tamanu Body Butter

Tamanu oil is great for dried and cracked skin. Combined with coconut oil, it brings about a rich, moisturizing body butter.

Ingredients

1 1/2 tsp Tamanu oil

1 cup coconut oil

10 drops essential oil of choice

Note:

Coconut oil is an excellent moisturizer, suitable for all skin types. It is rich in antioxidants and prevents the formation of free radicals. It can be used for face massage, for blemishes and other imperfections brought about by age or sun exposure.

It also acts as a gentle cleanser, especially in the eye area. It has antibacterial effect and can be used in the treatment of acne, small wounds, eczema and fungal infections.

Directions

1. Use a blender to mix all the ingredients until the mixture is fluffy.

2. Store in a dry, clean container, at room temperature.

Skin Toning Body Butter

Use this body butter on a daily basis to reduce stretch marks, scars and to tone your skin.

Ingredients

2 oz Shea butter

2 oz evening primrose oil

10 drops Jasmine essential oil

10 drops of Frankincense essential oil

Note:

Shea Butter is also a good moisturizer and sunscreen. It accelerates healing, soothes irritated skin, fights wrinkles and signs of aging. Additionally, it helps stretch marks, dermatitis as well as damaged dry hair and scalp.

Directions

1. Melt the Shea butter.

2. Add the primrose oil while the Shea butter is warm and mix well.

3. Put the mixture in the fridge and let cool until it begins to harden.

4. Add all the other ingredients and whisk with a hand mixer until smooth.

5. Store in a dry container.

Lavender Makeup Setting Spray

Ingredients:

5 drops of lavender essential oil

1 tablespoon aloe vera gel

2½ tablespoons purified water

1 tablespoon witch hazel

Directions:

1. Place the aloe vera gel into a jar and then add the witch hazel, blending well.

2. Add the lavender and water, mixing well

3. Pour it into a glass spray bottle carefully, shaking well.

4. Apply your makeup, and then hold the bottle a couple of inches away from the face. Mist your face with 1-2 pumps of your Lavender Make-up Setting.

5. Spray & air dry.

Essential Oil Blend For Baggy Eyes

Address those baggy eyes with lemon and lavender essentials oils, added to rosehip oil and aloe vera gel.

Ingredients:

1/2 ounce aloe vera gel

1/2 ounce rosehip seed oil

5 drops lemon essential oil

10 drops lavender essential oil

Note:

Rosehip oil helps your skin regenerate while Aloe vera works as a skin healer and anti-inflammatory agent.

Directions:

1. Combine all the ingredients in a glass spray bottle, shaking well.

2. Before bed, cleanse the face, remove all make-up then spray the solution onto the face (be sure to close your eyes!)

2. Massage gently under and around your eyes then leave to dry.

Stretch Mark Oil
Ingredients:

4 drops Rose

1 drop Rosemary

1/2 teaspoon Camellia Oil

1/2 teaspoon Sesame Oil

1/2 teaspoon Vitamin E Oil

1/2 teaspoon Wheat Germ Oil

Directions:

Massage on stretch mark areas.

Lush Body Oil

Ingredients:

4 oz Sunflower Oil

1 tsp Hazelnut Nut Oil

1 tsp Evening of Primrose Oil

1 tsp Macadamia Nut Oil

20 drops Vitamin E Oil

Directions:

1. Mix all ingredients together and store in a tightly covered bottle.

2. Refrigerate for longer shelf life.

Orange Chocolate Body Butter

This body butter is easy to prepare, it smells delicious too!

Ingredients

1/2 cup cocoa butter

1/2 cup coconut oil

20-40 drops Orange essential oil

Directions

1. Combine the coconut oil and the cocoa butter and the combination in a double boiler.

2. Place the mixture in the freezer until it starts to harden.

3. Add the essential oil and use a hand mixer to whip until it gets smooth.

4. Store the body butter in a glass jar.

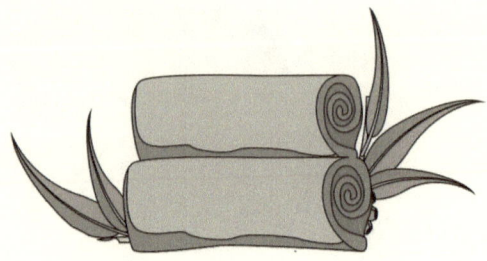

Homemade Sunburn Spray

A perfect sunburn remedy to also soothe inflammation and rehydrate the skin.

Ingredients:

10 drops lavender essential oil

10 drops peppermint essential oil

1/8 cup fractionated coconut oil

1/2 cup liquid aloe Vera juice

Directions:

1. Add 2 inches of water to a saucepan and place over medium heat.

2. Add coconut oil and aloe Vera juice in a jar. Place the jar in the saucepan and stir to liquefy and combine well.

3. Once combined, remove jar from sauce pan then add the oils to it, mixing well.

4. Pour into spray bottle. Store in a cool place.

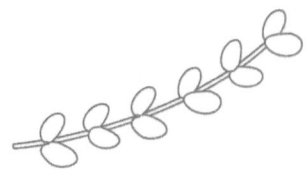

Soothing Body Butter

This body butter can be used for multiple purposes: as a deodorant, after shaving cream and to calm irritated skin.

Ingredients

6 tbsp cocoa butter

1/2 cup coconut oil

2 tbsp jojoba oil

15-20 drops tea tree oil

Directions

1. Use a double boiler to melt the cocoa butter.

2. Add the coconut and jojoba oil and mix well.

3. Cool the mixture in the fridge until it begins to harden.

4. Use a hand mixer to whip the mixture until it becomes smooth.

5. Add the tea tree oil and mix again.

6. Store in glass jar.

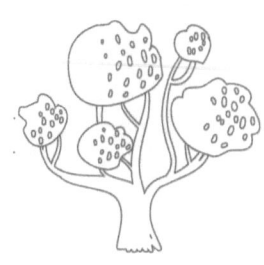

Spot Beater Oil

Ingredients:

1 oz Castor Oil

0.5 oz Emu Oil

30 drops Tea Tree Essential oil

Directions:

1. Mix together and then package.

2. Use oil as it easily soaks into skin.

Lime Coconut Body Butter

The perfect combination is for hot summer days.

Ingredients

1 tbsp olive oil

1/2 cup coconut oil

2 tbsp aloe Vera gel

20 drops lime essential oil

20 drops lemon essential oil

Directions

1. Combine all the ingredients.

2. Use a hand mixer to whisk until it gets the desired consistency.

3. Store in glass jar at room temperature.

Healing Body Butter

This body butter is great for dermatitis, stretch marks and skin rejuvenation.

Ingredients

1/2 cup cocoa butter

1/2 cup Shea butter

2 tbsp Rosehip oil

1 tbsp Argan Oil

10 drops of Frankincense essential oil

20 Drops Vanilla Extract

Directions

1. using a double boiler, melt the cocoa and Shea butter.

2. Let the mixture cool in the fridge until it begins to harden.

3. Add the other ingredients and use a hand mixer to whip the butter.

4. Store in a dry container.

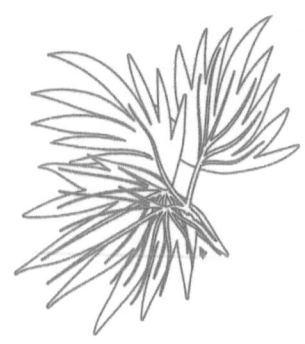

Anti Cellulite Body Butter

The ingredients used in this butter are helps to treat cellulite.

1/8 cup coconut oil

1/4 cup cocoa butter

1/8 cup sweet almond oil

20-30 drops Grapefruit essential oil

Directions

1. Combine the oils (save the essential oil) and melt in a double boiler on low.

2. Let the mixture rest in the freezer until it starts to solidify, about 20-25 minutes.

3. Add the essential oil and use a hand mixer to blend until it becomes smooth.

4. Store at room temperature for 6 months.

Sunscreen Lotion

Protect your skin from sunburn by using this all- natural sunscreen lotion.

Ingredients

1 oz cocoa butter

2 oz coconut oil

2 oz beeswax

1 oz Shea butter

2 oz avocado oil

10 drops carrot seed essential oil

1 Tbsp zinc oxide powder

25 drops Lavender essential oil

10 drops myrrh essential oil

2 drops Sandalwood essential oil

Directions

1. Combine the butters, oils and the beeswax in a jar.

2. Place the jar in a pan half filled with water and heat on low.

3. Once the ingredients melt, remove from heat.

4. Mix in the zinc oxide and stir carefully until well incorporated.

5. Add the essential oils and mix well. Store into a dry container.

Foot Lotion For Aching Feet

Ingredients:

1 tbsp Almond oil

1 tbsp Olive oil

1 tbsp Wheat germ oil

12 drops Eucalyptus essential oil

Directions:

1. Combine all ingredients in a bottle, shaking well.

2. Rub into the heels and feet.

3. Store in a cool dry place.

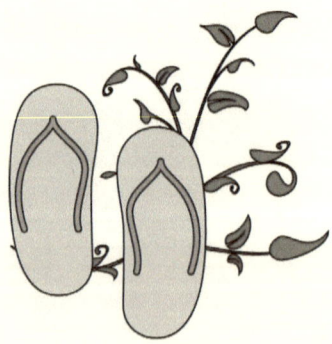

CREAMS
(Body creams, hand creams, eye creams, shaving creams & serums)

A natural skin care routine helps to achieve a smooth, healthy, blemish-free and translucent skin. Since natural oils are pure and free of toxic ingredients, they can safely and effectively be absorbed into the skin.

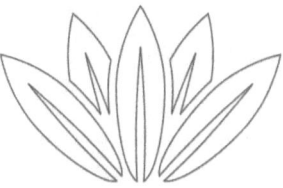

Recipes

Frankincense & Shea Butter Eye Cream
Moisturize your skin and the areas around your eyes with this recipe. It also helps to reduce the appearance of wrinkles.

Ingredients:

10 drops of frankincense essential oil

1 ounce Shea butter, unrefined

1 ounce aloe vera gel

1 ounce coconut oil, unrefined

½ teaspoon of vitamin E

Directions:

1. Combine all the ingredients in a small bowl.

2. Transfer to a glass jar and use around the eyes every morning and night.

3. This recipe can be used 30 times.

Beeswax Hand Cream

Ingredients:

¼ cup of Beeswax

¼ cup Almond oil

¼ cup of Honey

¼ cup of Vaseline petroleum jelly

¼ cup of Glycerin

2 tablespoon Liquid lecithin

3 drops Lavender essential oil

1 tablespoon of Bee pollen

Directions:

1. In a double boiler, melt together the petroleum jelly and beeswax.

2. Add the rest of the ingredients except essential oil and heat for 5 minutes until smooth.

3. Remove from heat and add the essential oil. While still hot, pour into a jar. It will harden as it cools.

4. Recipe makes about 1¼ cups.

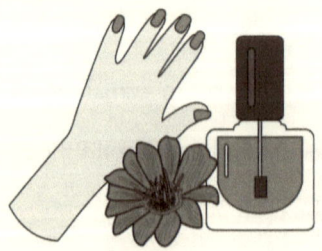

Homemade Shaving Cream

Hydrate and provide the essential vitamins that your skin requires with this awesome shaving cream. It is inexpensive and simple to make too!

Ingredients:

1/3 cup coconut oil

15 drops lavender oil

1/3 cup Shea butter

2 tbsp olive oil

Directions:

1. Melt Shea butter and coconut oil in a small saucepan over low-medium heat.

2. Once it melts, remove from heat and put in a bowl.

3. Add the oils and refrigerate until solid.

4. Remove and whip 3 to 4 minutes until fluffy. Shaving cream can be used 30 times.

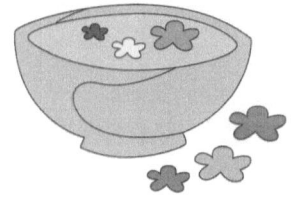

Rose Beeswax Hand Cream

Ingredients:

¼ cup of beeswax

¼ cup of coconut oil

3 tablespoon baby oil

3 drops Rosewood essential oil

1/3 cup Glycerin

Directions:

1. In a double boiler, melt together the petroleum jelly and beeswax.

2. Add the rest of the ingredients except essential oil and heat for 5 minutes until smooth.

3. Remove from heat and add the essential oil. While still hot, pour into a jar. It will harden as it cools.

4. Recipe makes about 1 cup.

Bee Pollen Hand Cream

Ingredients:

1/2 cup petroleum jelly

1/2 cup glycerin

1/3 cup beeswax

2 tablespoons of bee pollen

3 drops Lavender essential oil

Directions:

1. In a double boiler, melt together the petroleum jelly and beeswax.

2. Add the glycerin and then heat for a few minutes until the mixture is well heated. Add the bee pollen and essential oil.

3. While still hot, pour into a jar. It will harden as it cools.

4. Recipe makes about 1¼ cups.

Lemon Facial Cleansing Cream
Ingredients:

1 tbsp Beeswax

3 tbsp Jojoba oil or Coconut oil

1 tbsp Witch hazel

1 tbsp Lemon juice

1/8 tsp Bicarbonate of soda

6 drops Lemon essential oil

Directions:

1. In a saucepan, melt the beeswax over low heat. Add the coconut oil (or jojoba) and beat for 5 minutes with a hand mixer.

2. Heat the witch hazel and lemon juice in another saucepan until warm. Add in the bicarbonate of soda to dissolve.

3. Add this liquid mixture to the cream, beat until well combined. Leave the cream to cool for a while.

4. Add the lemon essential oil and spoon into a container.

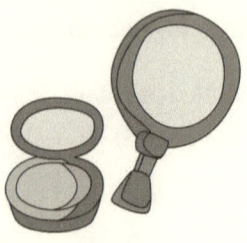

Beeswax Cold Cream

Ingredients:

1/3 cup Beeswax

1/3 cup Glycerin

1 tbsp Liquid lecithin

¼ cup baby oil

¼ cup Almond oil

1 tbsp Bee pollen

3drops Essential oil of choice

Directions:

1. Melt beeswax over a double boiler.

2. Add the rest of the ingredients, except essential oil and heat until smooth then add the essential oil.

3. While still hot, pour into a container. It will harden as it cools.

4. Recipe makes about 1½ cups.

Rash Cream With Aloe & Lavender

Ingredients:

¼ cup cocoa butter

¼ cup cup grapeseed oil

2 tablespoons aloe vera gel

2 tablespoons bentonite clay

1-2 tablespoons witch hazel

10 drops lavender essential oil

Directions:

1. Place the grapeseed oil and cocoa butter in a double boiler pan and melt on low heat, stirring well.

2. Add the aloe vera gel and keep stirring. Remove from heat.

3. Now add the witch hazel, bentonite clay, and lavender, stirring until well blended. Transfer to a glass jar with a tight-fitting lid.

4. Apply to the skin two times a day; let it dry for about 15 minutes then rinse off with warm water and a washcloth

5. This recipe: 4–5 ounces.

Beeswax Almond Hand Cream

Ingredients:

¼ cup beeswax

½ cup almond oil

½ cup coconut oil

¼ cup rosewater

3 drops Essential oil of choice

Directions:

1. Melt the coconut oil and beeswax over a double boiler. Add the remaining ingredients

2. Add the rest of the ingredients, except essential oil and heat until smooth then add the essential oil.

3. While still hot, pour into a container. It will harden as it cools. This makes about 1½ cups.

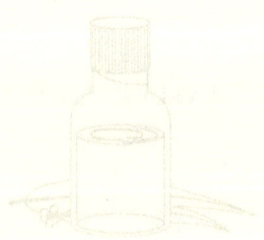

Heavy Duty Hand Cream

Ingredients:

2 tbsp Shaved beeswax

1/2 tsp carnuba wax

2 tbsp Jojoba oil

1 tsp Aloe Vera gel

10 drops Vitamin E oil 4 or Vitamin E capsules

1 drop any essential oil

Directions:

1. Melt the beeswax, carnuba wax, Jojoba oil and Aloe Vera in a pot.

2. Remove from heat, beat until cool and add Vitamin E oil before the mixture thickens.

3. Continue beating until mixture becomes creamy then add essential oil and keep beating until cream has totally cooled.

4. Spoon cream into a jar and store in a cool dark place.

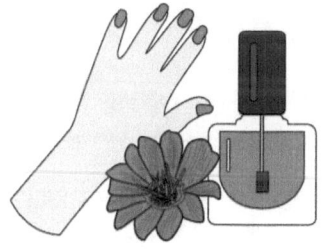

DIY Stretch Mark Cream

Stretch marks with their scarred appearance can be embarrassing. Typically found on the hips, thighs, breasts, abdomen, and upper arms and lower back; stretch marks with their glossy and streaked looks can be eliminated using this recipe which makes 6–8 ounces.

Ingredients:

3/4 ounce unrefined cocoa butter

3 ounces unrefined coconut oil

¾ oz unrefined shea butter

6 tablespoons water

3 tablespoons sweet almond oil

2 teaspoons vitamin E oil

20 drops cypress essential oil

20 drops lavender essential oil

10 drops grapefruit essential oil

10 drops helichrysum essential oil

Directions:

1. Melt the almond oil, cocoa butter, coconut oil and shea butter in a sauce pan very low heat.

2. Add melted mixture to water until smooth and combined.

3. Remove from heat but keep mixing until mixture cools to room temperature and develops a creamy consistency.

4. Now stir in the lavender, helichrysum, grapefruit and cypress essential oils, together with the vitamin E oil.

5. Store the cream in a dark glass container.

Homemade Anti-Aging Serum

Do away with expensive anti aging serums that are filled with harmful chemicals. This all- natural anti aging serum recipe is loaded with nutrients as well as antioxidants that will rejuvenate your skin.

Ingredients:

1/2 tablespoon Jojoba Oil

20 drops of frankincense or lavender oil

1/2 tablespoon Evening Primrose Oil

1/2 tablespoon pomegranate oil

10 drops of Carrot Seed Oil

15 drops Vitamin E oil

Directions:

1. Combine all the ingredients in a dark glass bottle.

2. Use on face, neck and chest every morning and night.

Eye Serum For Dark Circles &Puffiness

Reduce dark circles and eye puffiness within a few days with this recipe.

Ingredients:

1/2 ounce rosehip seed oil

1/2 ounce aloe vera gel

5 drops lemon essential oil

10 drops lavender essential oil

Directions:

1. Combine all ingredients in a glass spray bottle and shake well.

2. Before bed, cleanse the face, remove all make-up and spray the solution onto the face. (Be sure to close your eyes).

3. Massage the solution gently under and around your eyes and let it dry.

Note: Rosehip oil is rich in essential fatty acids which help with tissue regeneration. It also contains lots of vitamins that helps to protect the skin. Lavender and lemon essential oil contains powerful antioxidants and helps nourish the skin.

Moisturizing Anti-Aging Face Cream
Ingredients:

4 tsp Beeswax

4 tbsp Olive oil

2tbsp Shea butter, coconut oil or mango butter

8 tbsp Water or green tea

1 tbsp Jojoba

1 tbsp Glycerin

10- 15 drops Essential oil

Directions:

1. Melt the beeswax and oil in a double boiler. Stir until well mixed. Add the shear butter; stir until it well melted into the wax.

2. Remove from the heat and then whip with a hand-held mixer while adding the aloe Vera, green tea and glycerin.

3. Continue whipping until the cream becomes light and fluffy. Leave it to cool to room temperature.

4. Blend in the essential oil, stir until fully combined. Pour into a container and seal.

5. This recipe makes about 227g of anti-aging face cream.

Note:

Since this recipe contains no preservative, keep unused cream refrigerated for about 6 months. Alternatively, keep in a cool place for about 3 months.

Remove cream from container, using washable or cosmetic spatulas and not your fingers to prevent contamination.

Witch Hazel Eye Solution
Get rid of those bags under your eyes when you wake up.

Ingredients:

10 drops of lavender essential oil

1/2 oz of witch hazel extract

1/2 oz of pure aloe vera gel

10 drops chamomile essential oil

Directions:

1. Add all the ingredients to a small lidded glass jar and blend.

2. Let it chill overnight.

3. Upon waking, apply a little amount of the solution around the eyes. Let it sit for several hours before removing.

4. This solution will last 20 uses.

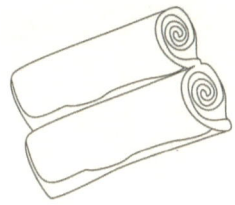

PERFUMES RECIPES

(Perfumes, solid perfumes, colognes & aftershaves)

Perfume making is easy, fun and extremely economical. It is also organic and natural, keeping you safe from harmful chemical ingredients contained in store-bought products. Perfume comprises three major ingredients: essential oils, water and pure grain alcohol. However, essential oils are the most crucial ingredient needed for perfume making.

While making perfumes, try not to smell too many essential oils at once so your nose does not become overworked, otherwise you will find it difficult to distinguish one scent from another. But if this happens, simply hold fresh coffee beans a few inches away from your nose and inhale a number of times. Your nose will get back to business in no time!

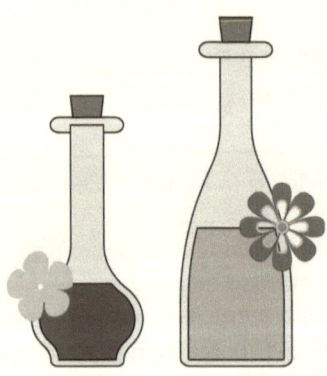

10 Helpful Tips For Perfume Making

1. The higher the number of essential oil drops used, the stronger the perfume.

2. Do not substitute tap water for distilled water.

3. For a little color in your perfume, use only natural vegetable food dye.

4. The longer a perfume sit, the stronger the scent and the more it will last.

5. Apply solid perfume moderately on business cards. This smells great!

6. For your perfume to blend well and settle, it may take between 1-3 months; so shake the bottle every day.

7. Store perfume in a dark bottle or glass container to make it last longer.

8. For each essential oil applied, use a separate pipette otherwise wash it in alcohol after each use. This helps to keeps your perfume from being marred or contaminated.

9. For a higher incense fragrance in your perfume, add 2-3 drops of Ambrette Seed, Cedar Moss, Copal, Tonka Bean or Benzoin resin. They act as fixatives and can therefore offer a stronger and long-lasting perfume. However, use them moderately because they have strong effects.

10. Experiment for more luxurious scents.

Whispering Drops Perfume

Ingredients:

2 cups distilled water

3tbsp Vodka

5 drops Sandalwood essential oil

10 drops Bergamot essential oil

10 drops Cassis essential oil

Note:

Vodka serves as perfect carrier oil. It is odorless, enhances the fragrance of the perfume and sustains its durability

Directions:

1. Combine all the ingredients together, shaking well.

2. Let it settle for 12 hours then store in a cool dry area.

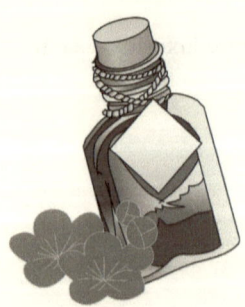

Rich Spicy Cologne

Ingredients

1 fluid ounce vodka

3 fluid ounces water

8 drops bay essential oil

11 drops bergamot essential oil

2 drops neroli essential oil

3 drops vetiver essential oil

Directions

1. Mix the alcohol, essential oils and water in a glass bottle.

2. Allow the mixture to sit for 2-6 weeks. Shake to mix occasionally.

3. Wear and enjoy.

Fiery Passions Perfume

This perfume has a sensual and exotic aroma that you can't help but love.

Ingredients

3 drops Neroli essential oil

2 drops ylang ylang essential oil

3 drops passionflower essential oil

1/2 pt (300ml) 70% vodka

Directions

1. Pour the vodka into a dark bottle.

2. Add other ingredients and mix thoroughly.

3. Let the mixture settle for 1 week in a cool and dry area.

4. Dab on pulse points and enjoy your fiery passion perfume.

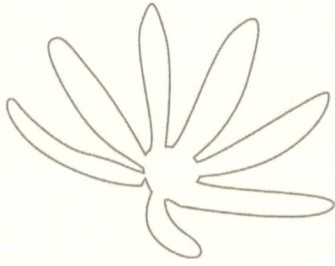

Musky floral Perfume Blend

This perfume blend can be used on its own or use as a musk oil alternative to add to other blends.

Ingredients

7 drops myrrh essential oil

9 drops patchouli essential oil

7 drops cedarwood essential oil

9 drops frankincense essential oil

10 drops Vanilla Essentials

1 fluid ounce of carrier oil

Note:

Patchouli oil is a wonderful choice for a women's perfume or even a man's cologne. Since it does not evaporate quickly, it is generally used as a fixative. It will also prolong the scent in your perfume.

Directions

1. Combine all oils.

2. Let it sit for 3- 7days, mixing occasionally.

Fruitwood Perfume

Fruitwood perfume is a citrusy scent. The verbena and lemongrass adds to it a woodsy fragrance (generally loved by men).

Ingredients

5 drops of neroli oil

5 tsp vodka

1/2 tsp distilled water

10 drops lemongrass essential oil

10 drops of grapefruit oil

15 drops lemon essential oil

3 drops of cedarwood oil

2 drops benzoin oil

10 drops verbena essential oil

Directions

1. Pour the vodka into a dark bottle.

2. Add other ingredients and mix thoroughly.

3. Let the mixture settle for 2-3 weeks in a cool and dry area, shaking and inverting bottle occasionally to blend the scent.

4. Dab on pulse points and enjoy your Victorian scent.

Exotic Perfume Blend

Ingredients

2 drops palmarosa essential oil

3 drops bergamot essential oil

4 drops sandalwood essential oil

3 drops rose absolute essential oil

½ fluid ounce vodka or any high-proof grain alcohol

Directions

1. Mix the alcohol and essential oils in a glass bottle.

2. Let it sit for 2 to 6 weeks. Shake to mix occasionally.

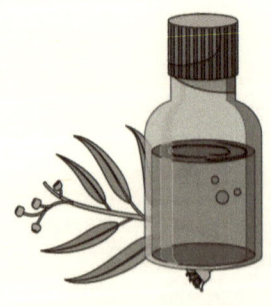

Soothing Body Perfume

Ingredients:

25 drops Sandalwood

3 drops Rose, Jasmine or Neroli

2 tbsp Jojoba

Directions:

1. Blend all the oils together then store in an airtight dark-colored glass jar.

2. Leave for some days to mature.

3. Dab only a drop onto your pulse points.

4. Use sparingly due to the heavy concentration of essential oils.

<u>Note</u>:

Jojoba oil is great choice for base oil. It is waxy, non-greasy, easily absorbable oil made from jojoba seeds. It has an extensive shelf-life as well.

Summer Sweet Perfume

This relaxing and warm blend is extremely valuable during the dark winter months.

Ingredients

10 drops Lavender essential oil

1 drop Cedarwood essential oil

5 drops Chamomile essential oil

1 drop Geranium essential oil

4 drops Cardamom essential oil

1 tsp organic Jojoba Oil

Directions

1. Drip all the essential oils into a glass bottle.

2. Roll the bottle between palms to mix the oils evenly

3. Add Jojoba oil and roll again.

4. If you want a stronger perfume, add more essential oils

<u>**Note:**</u>

Geranium oil emits a rosy and delicate fragrance and is usually used to reduce fatigue, treat anxiety and stress. Similar in properties to Rose essential oil, it is a cheaper alternative and provides harmony and balance.

Homemade Deodorant For Men
Ingredients:

50 ml Vodka

50 ml Pure witch hazel

15 drops Sandalwood

5 drops Black pepper

10 drops Cypress

5 drops Frankincense

5 drops Tea tree

Directions:

1. Add the oils into your glass bottle

2. Add the vodka and witch hazel.

3. Close firmly with the sprayer and cap.

4. Shake thoroughly before each use so as to redistribute the oils.

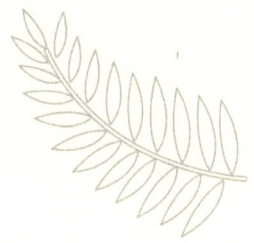

Midnight Garden
Ingredients

2 tablespoons jojoba oil

15 drops clove oil

6 drops cedarwood oil

9 drops lavender oil

2 1/2 tablespoons spring or distilled water

6 tablespoons vodka

Directions

1. Place the carrier oil into a curing bottle.

2. Add the essential oils.

3. Add the vodka, place lid on bottle and shake vigorously for some minutes.

4. Let the bottle sit for 2 to 6 weeks. Check the scent regularly.

5. Once you are pleased with it, add the water to the blend. Shake for 1 minute.

6. Get a funnel; place a coffee filter into it and then transfer contents from the curing bottle to a storing bottle.

7. Label and wear.

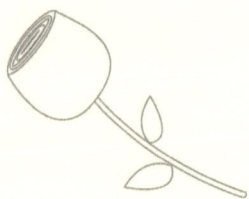

Love Tonic Perfume
Increase your love feelings of love with this pleasant aphrodisiac

Ingredients

15 drops bergamot essential oil

2 drops vanilla essential oil

3 drops sandalwood essential oil

3 drops cedar-wood essential oil

300ml 70% vodka or alcohol

Directions

1. Pour the vodka or any other kind of alcohol into a jar or bottle.

2. Add the oils, shaking well to mix.

3. Set aside for 1 week before using.

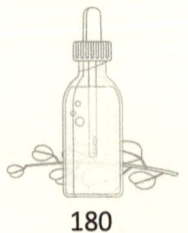

This blend smells great! It is uplifting and comforting as well.

Ingredients

1 tsp organic Jojoba Oil

4 drops Spruce essential oil

2 drops Cedarwood essential oil

2 drops Fir Needle essential oil

1 drop Bergamot essential oil

1 drop Vetiver essential oil

Directions

1. Drip all the essential oils into a glass bottle.

2. Roll the bottle between palms to mix the oils evenly

3. Add Jojoba oil and roll again.

4. If you want a stronger perfume, add more essential oils

Surprise Perfume

This amazing fragrance will certainly inspire admiration, awe and wonder.

Ingredients

10 drops rosemary essential oil

10 drops cypress essential oil

2 cups distilled water

5 drops St. John's wort

3 tablespoons vodka

Directions

1. Mix together all ingredients in a dark color bottle, shake well.

2. Let it settle for 12-18 hours. Store it in a cool & dry area.

3. Dab on pulse points.

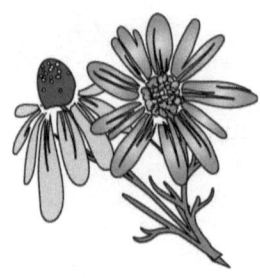

Tangerine -Patchouli Solid Perfume
For half-ounce pot of solid perfume

Ingredients

40 drops Tangerine Essential Oil

50 drops Patchouli Essential Oil

5 grams Beeswax

15 ml Jojoba Oil

Directions:

1. In a small shot glass, measure out the jojoba oil.

2. Add essential oils and blend well.

3. Measure out the beeswax. Place it in a small glass and heat it in a water bath until it is melted

4. Remove from the heat but keep the melted beeswax container in the hot water.

5. Pour the essential oil mixture into the melted beeswax.

6. Pour the melted perfume quickly and carefully into a container and leave to harden for about 30 minutes.

7. Label and enjoy.

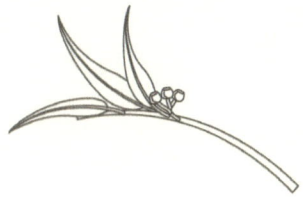

Citrus Cologne

A revitalizing and stimulating aroma made from fresh citrus.

Ingredients

1 fresh Grapefruit peel, zest only

1 fresh Lemon peel, zest only

Basil, Chamomile, Lavender or Peppermint essential oils

8 oz Vodka

Directions

1. In a glass mason jar, combine the grapefruit and lemon peel zest.

2. Add the vodka until it rises above the peel zest by 1-2 inches.

3. Cap it tightly and shake 2-3 times daily.

4. Leave for 2 to 6 weeks then strain the citrus peels out and pour cologne into a glass bottle.

5. Add 2 drops essential oil per 1 tablespoon of finished cologne.

6. If you want stronger cologne, add more essential oil.

Alpha Male Cologne

Ingredients

15 drops Mandarin or Bergamot

5 drops Bay Laurel

2.5 oz. High Proof Vodka

1 oz. Distilled Water

15 drops Patchouli

3 drops Black Pepper or Ginger

2-3 drops Vetiver or 5 drops Oakmoss Absolute

1-2 drops of Neroli (optional)

Directions:

1. Combine water and alcohol and add to a 4 oz. glass bottle with a sprayer top. Add the oils, shaking well.

2. Let it rest for 5-7days, shaking the bottle twice a day for the oils to blend.

3. Shake the cologne thoroughly before each use. First test it by applying it to a small area in your forearm before fully using.

Homemade Oil Aftershave

While this is not cologne, it is long-lasting and smells great.

Ingredients

5 drops Coriander essential oil

6 drops Bergamot essential oil

1 drop Cedarwood essential oil

3 drops Sandalwood essential oil

4 drops Neroli essential oil

10 ml Jojoba Oil

Directions

1. Pour the jojoba oil in a mixing container.

2. Carefully add the essential oils to it one by one. Mix well.

3. Pour the mixture into small glass container, seal and leave for1 a week.

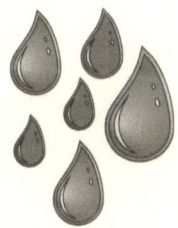

Timeout Blend
Ingredients

40 drops lavender Essential Oil

50 drops geranium Essential Oil

5 grams Beeswax

15 ml Jojoba Oil

Directions:

1. in a small shot glass, measure out the jojoba oil.

2. Add essential oils and blend well.

3. Measure out the beeswax. Place it in a small glass and heat it in a water bath until it is melted

4. Remove from the heat but keep the melted beeswax container in the hot water.

5. Pour the essential oil mixture into the melted beeswax.

6. Pour the melted perfume quickly and carefully into a container and leave to harden for about 30 minutes.

7. Label and enjoy.

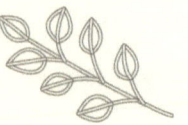

Citrus Lavender Solid Perfume

Ingredients

12 drops sweet orange essential oil

12 drops lemon essential oil

12 drops lavender essential oil

12 drops bergamot essential oil

2 tsp beeswax

2 tsp carrier oil – jojoba or sweet almond oil

Directions:

1. Blend the Essential Oils in a cup

 2. In another cup, add two teaspoons of almond or jojoba oil.

3. Melt the Beeswax in a pot.

4. Add the Carrier Oil, stir until combined.

5. Remove from heat and add essential oils quickly, stirring until just combined.

6. Pour into container, cover and leave to set for about 10 minutes. Enjoy!

The End